D1644679

The British School of Osteopathy

* 3 3 0 3 *

THE BACK
RELIEF FROM PAIN

Dr Alan Stoddard is both a physician as well as an eminent osteopath. For twenty-six years he was consultant in charge of the physical medicine department of a hospital near London. He was a member of the Board of Governors of the British School of Osteopathy where he lectures regularly. His two earlier books, *A Manual of Osteopathic Technique* and *A Manual of Osteopathic Practice*, are now classic osteopathic textbooks and have been published and reprinted throughout the world.

Dr Stoddard runs a busy osteopathic practice. He and his wife live by the sea and have six grown-up children. He swims every day, likes gardening and sailing in his boat when he gets time.

To all back sufferers

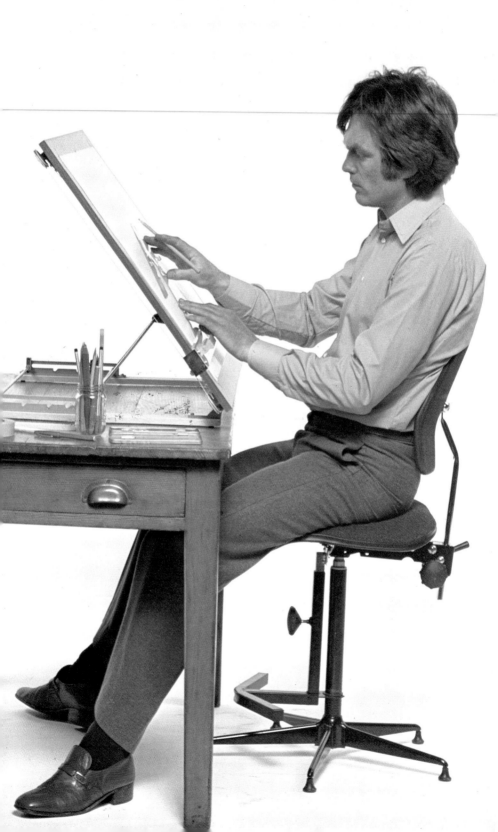

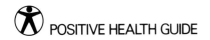

POSITIVE HEALTH GUIDE

THE BACK
RELIEF FROM PAIN

Patterns of back pain –
how to deal with and avoid them.

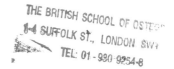
Alan Stoddard

MB, BS, DO, DPhys Med

MARTIN DUNITZ

© **Dr Alan Stoddard 1979**
Second Edition 1980
Third, revised edition 1981
Reprinted 1982
Reprinted 1983
Reprinted 1984
Reprinted 1986

First published in Great Britain in 1979 by
Martin Dunitz Ltd, 154 Camden High
Street, London NW1 0NE
This revised edition published 1981

Studio photographs by Bill Ling
Location photographs by Simon Farrell
Cover photograph of Malcolm Stoddard
who played Darwin in the BBC
Television –Time Life series 'The Voyage of
The Beagle'.

**British Library Cataloguing in
Publication Data**

Stoddard, Alan
    The back, relief from pain.
    (Positive health guides).
    1. Backache
    I. Title   II. Series
    616.7'3'06 RD768

ISBN 0-906348-26-9 paperback

Printed by Toppan Printing Company (S) Pte Ltd, Singapore

CONTENTS

INTRODUCTION

If you suffer from back pain the first step towards relieving it is to understand the nature of the pain and what has caused it. If you know what is happening to your back, the pain will be much less worrying. Is the pain temporary or permanent? Is it likely to recur and what effect is it going to have on your livelihood, your hobbies, your garden, your golf? These are the sort of questions which need answering.

My purpose in writing this book is to present a practical guide to back pain and to offer relief for all back-pain sufferers. The book is designed to explain all the causes of back pain and to show how these causes affect the anatomy and physiology of the spine and how, through the nervous system, they affect the body as a whole. The patterns of back pain are described to help you understand what is wrong. At the same time, I give practical suggestions and exercises to help you relieve the pain, whether it is a sudden, totally incapacitating pain or a slow dull ache that always seems to be with you. I outline methods of treatment currently available to enable you to seek advice in the right direction. Finally, you may find that by making sometimes minor adaptations or adjustments to your way of life, as described, the persistence or recurrence of your back pain could be dramatically reduced.

While the book is directed primarily towards the general reader I hope that it will be useful to workers in the field of spinal pain. I have attempted to steer a middle course between over-simplification and too much technical detail and have tried to use non-technical language, but some terms are unavoidable and you will soon learn these words.

It has been estimated by the Arthritis and Rheumatism Council of Great Britain that about twenty million working days each year are lost by the employed population of this country because of back pain. Statistics are similar in other Western countries. These figures deal only with employed people and do not take into account the days of incapacity suffered by wives and others not on the employment register, nor of the misery of backache suffered by men and women who struggle on with their normal duties despite back pain. About half the patients who attend doctors for back problems are women and only a fifth of these are included in the employed list, so that the official figures understate the size of the problem. The average absence from work is thirty-three days for patients on the sick list with back problems. If the average time away from work is about five weeks this implies that the severe cases are incapacitated for much longer.

Some people are permanently restricted in work and sport. For the majority of back sufferers, however, the problem is a nuisance rather than an incapacity and most people are free of back trouble most of the time; but there must be few, if any, people who have never, at any stage in their lives, had some back pain. Our backs, therefore, assume great importance in all our lives and any method or system which helps to reduce back pain is worthwhile.

The causes of back pain

Back pain is caused, broadly, by physical strains known as mechanical strains and stresses and their after-effects; it is also caused by deteriorating changes, known as degenerative changes, in the vertebrae, discs and other parts of the spine. Pain may also arise from disease of the spine and from psychological factors. All these basic causes can be influenced by heredity, occupational hazards, injuries in sport, on the road and in the home. Other factors include pregnancies, bad posture while standing, walking, bending, sitting and lying down, unbalanced diet and nutrition, and anxieties about the pain. The cossetted life of soft beds, soft armchairs, soft car seats, and the effect of poor muscles from disuse or unaccustomed use, can lead to back pain.

Popular misconceptions

There are many misconceptions about back pain – including the following:

1. All back pain is due to slipped discs.

2. Because a patient has had a bad back he will always have one.

3. Slipped discs always manifest in the same way.

4. The whole disc displaces.

5. Osteopaths are wizards and can cure back pain with one quick click.

6. Manipulation is necessarily painful.

7. Corsets are a waste of time and should never be used.

8. Disc trouble will lead to arthritis.

9. Lumbago is something funny.

10. A normal spinal X-ray means that there is nothing wrong with the spine.

None of these assertions is true though there may be a grain of truth here and there.

1 THE SPINE

If you want practical advice and are not interested in underlying causes for your back problem you may wish to skip the next two chapters. An understanding of the structure and workings of the spine, however, will help you to cope with it and to accept advice or treatment which you may be offered.

Anatomy of the spine

The spine consists of a series of vertebrae attached together by ligaments. It could be compared with the mast of a sailing boat which is supported by stays and shrouds corresponding to the ligaments. The vertebrae are separated from each other by discs of cartilage. Attached to the spine are the ribs, the limbs and the skull by more ligaments and muscles (fig. 1).

Each vertebra has bony processes (or protuberances) which project backwards and sideways for the attachment of muscles and ligaments. These processes, jutting out from the back of the vertebral body, join together to form a circle – the vertebral canal through which the spinal cord runs. The processes are marked on fig. 4. They are called pedicles, laminae, transverse and spinous processes.

Between the vertebral arch above and the vertebral arch below are spaces called foramina through which spinal nerves pass. One large and several smaller nerves emerge from each side of the spinal cord to run through these foramina. The nerves spread out round the body and supply virtually all the tissues of the body. A rare exception of tissue which does not have a nerve supply is the intervertebral disc.

On each side of the vertebra are the intervertebral joints. These are small joints and are similar in construction to all other joints in the body. They are called apophyseal joints. They help and influence movement between adjacent vertebrae.

It will be seen from the illustrations of the spine, looking from the *front* (fig. 2), that there is a gradual increase in size of vertebrae from the top downwards. The design of each vertebra is modified according to its workload.

The neck (cervical) vertebrae, of which there are seven, are relatively small because they merely support the weight of the head which averages 12 lb (5 kg).

The chest (thoracic) vertebrae serve for the attachment of ribs and this area is relatively inflexible because the rib cage prevents much movement. There are twelve ribs on each side attached to the twelve thoracic vertebrae. All mammals have seven cervical vertebrae but not necessarily twelve thoracic vertebrae. Even

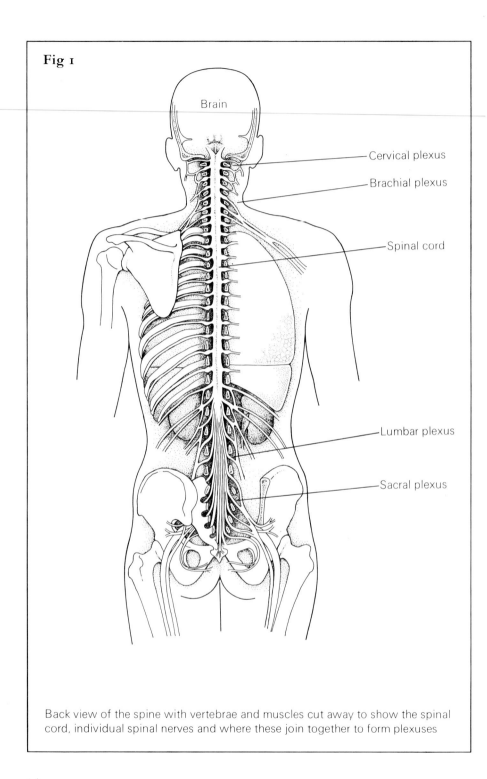

Fig 1

Brain

Cervical plexus

Brachial plexus

Spinal cord

Lumbar plexus

Sacral plexus

Back view of the spine with vertebrae and muscles cut away to show the spinal cord, individual spinal nerves and where these join together to form plexuses

the whale, which does not look as if it has a neck at all, and the giraffe, which looks as if it might have twenty vertebrae, both have only seven cervical vertebrae In the human it is possible to get an extra rib attached to the last cervical vertebra and sometimes the twelfth rib is missing.

There are normally five loin (lumbar) vertebrae but occasionally four or even six. The lumbar vertebrae are larger because not only do they have to support the weight of the head, arms and trunk, but they are fairly mobile and they have to withstand enormous leverages. The last lumbar vertebra joins the spine to the pelvis at the sacrum, or triangular bone at the back of the pelvis.

The pelvis (fig. 5) consists of three bones which form a joint in front and two joints behind called sacro-iliac joints. Small movements are possible at these joints especially in women during childbirth, but after thirty years of age in men and fifty years in women the mobility of these joints virtually ceases by fibrous union and loss of elasticity in the ligaments.

The normal spine when viewed either from in front or behind is straight and any deviation to the left or right indicates some mechanical disorder.

The *side* view of the normal spine (fig. 2) shows gentle curves forward in the neck, backward in the thoracic area and forward in the lumbar area. The sacrum has a small convexity in front to help shape the pelvis which contains the rectum, bladder and genital organs. This convexity serves to accommodate a baby's head towards the end of a pregnancy.

The tail or coccyx which is attached to the lower end of the sacrum has three or four segments and is normally only about 1 in (2.5 cm) long. Wagging your tail is not feasible! But each time you contract your pelvic floor muscles when opening the bowels or bladder or during sexual intercourse there are small movements of the coccyx. If such movements are restricted as a result of injury, you may notice that the coccyx becomes painful when sitting or in any of the activities mentioned above.

If the forward and backward curves of the spine are altered (either an increase or decrease of the curves), this strains the ligaments and sometimes causes pain. A hollow back is called a lordosis (page 43) and a prominent thoracic spine (or 'rounded shoulders') is called a kyphosis (page 47).

The foramina on each side in the *neck* (fig. 4) are not merely holes but channels formed by the transverse processes which are U-shaped when seen from the side. This provides support and protection for the spinal nerves as they emerge from the spinal cord. The transverse processes also have holes in them to transmit arteries and veins in a vertical direction. Although well protected the nerves, arteries and veins are vulnerable by the sheer complexity of the anatomy in the region of the foramina. The foramina are bounded in front by the disc, above and below by the laminae and behind by the small apophyseal joints. The size of a foramen is ample, when normal, for transmitting the nerves and blood vessels, but if a piece of disc displaces or if the apophyseal joint swells then the foramen is reduced in size and this can compress either the nerves or the blood vessels or both.

15

Fig 2

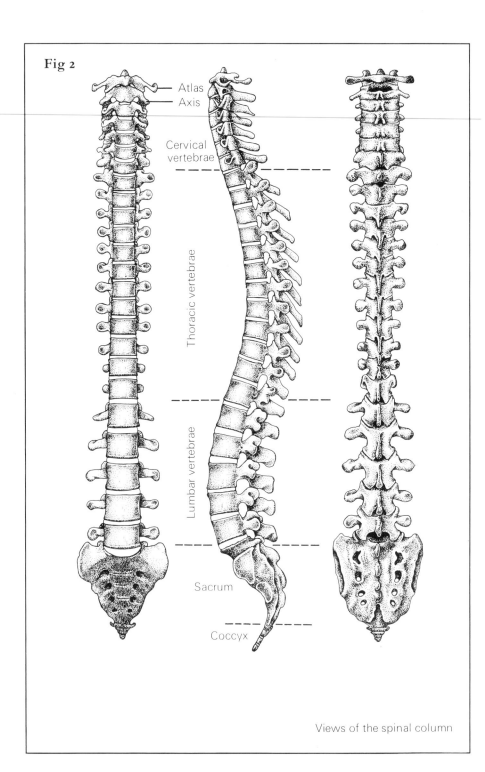

Atlas
Axis
Cervical vertebrae
Thoracic vertebrae
Lumbar vertebrae
Sacrum
Coccyx

Views of the spinal column

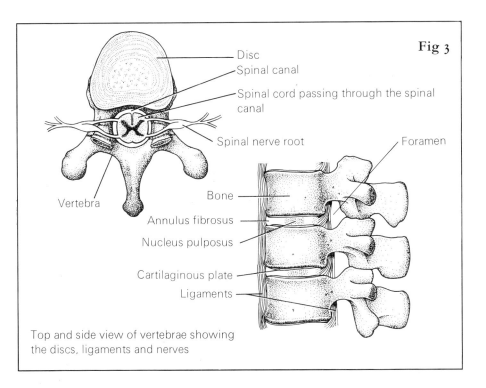

Disc
Spinal canal
Spinal cord passing through the spinal canal
Spinal nerve root
Foramen
Bone
Vertebra
Annulus fibrosus
Nucleus pulposus
Cartilaginous plate
Ligaments

Fig 3

Top and side view of vertebrae showing the discs, ligaments and nerves

The foramina in the *thoracic* spine are large and, as the discs there are subjected to less stress, there are fewer problems in this area compared with the neck and lumbar areas. The nerves which emerge through the foramina pass round the body to supply the ribs, muscles and skin of the chest and abdomen. Sometimes pain is felt in front of the chest and in the abdomen as a result of pressure on the thoracic nerves in the spine. This can cause confusion for both the doctor and for you because such pain suggests that something is wrong with the heart or lungs or stomach or bowel whereas the pain is spinal in origin.

The foramina in the *lumbar* spine (fig. 3) are very large above, but the last two are smaller especially the one between the fifth lumbar vertebra and sacrum. Curiously enough this foramen transmits the largest in size of the lumbar nerves. Consequently, small disc protrusions or small swellings of the apophyseal joints in the lower lumbar levels cause as much nerve pressure as do large protrusions in the upper lumbar area. Another reason why the lowest two vertebrae and discs are more vulnerable to stress is that this is where the flexible spine meets the rigid pelvis and where maximum leverage occurs.

It would be helpful in describing the spine to point out the differences between muscles, tendons, ligaments and cartilages.

Muscles have the power to contract and their function is to move bones to which they are attached. For example, the biceps muscle has the power to bend the elbow. A secondary function, but often just as important, is to act as a

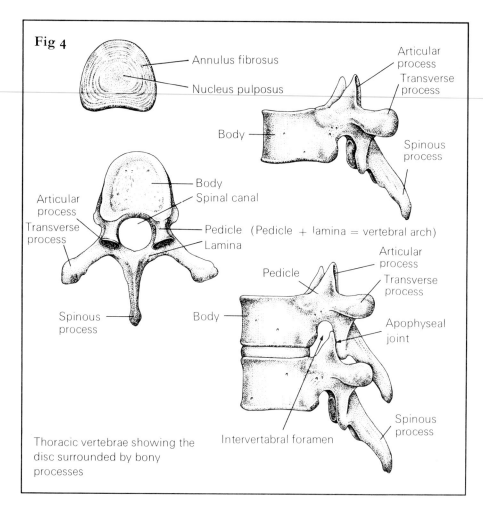

Fig 4

Annulus fibrosus

Nucleus pulposus

Articular process

Transverse process

Body

Spinous process

Body

Spinal canal

Articular process

Transverse process

Pedicle   (Pedicle + lamina = vertebral arch)

Lamina

Spinous process

Body

Articular process

Transverse process

Pedicle

Apophyseal joint

Spinous process

Thoracic vertebrae showing the disc surrounded by bony processes

Intervertabral foramen

stabilizing influence to keep one section of the body firm while moving another part. The back muscles have a lot of work to do in stabilizing the trunk for the limbs to act upon. Each time you contract your biceps, the shoulder muscles are holding firm while the arm takes the strain of the movement and the back muscles contract to keep your balance while your arm lifts the weight. Muscles are thick in the middle and thin near their attachments to the bones and in some places the thin ends become *tendons* or leaders.

Where bones join together joints are formed and the ends of the bones are kept together by ligaments.

Ligaments are semi-elastic structures but there is a definite limit to their elasticity and when forced beyond that limit they tear and become painful as, for example, with a sprained ankle. Ligaments also protest if they are stretched to their elastic limit and are kept so stretched for prolonged periods. These ligaments then gradually elongate under the stretch and cause pain. A good

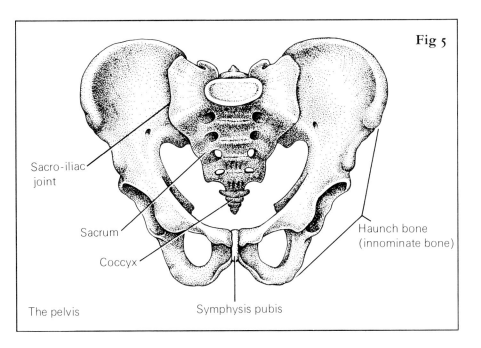

Fig 5

Sacro-iliac joint

Sacrum

Coccyx

Haunch bone
(innominate bone)

The pelvis

Symphysis pubis

example of this is found in the feet. A walker does not get flat feet because the foot ligaments are stretched intermittently, whereas a shopkeeper gets flat feet because of continuous stretch on the foot ligaments while standing still for long periods. They lengthen and the arch drops. A similar process occurs in the spine as will be explained later.

The opposing surfaces of the bones which form joints are covered by *cartilage*. This cartilage helps movement. All movable joints have such cartilage and some joints, like the knee, have additional pieces for their cushioning effect. In the spine this cartilage is called a disc and each disc intervenes between one vertebra and the next.

Discs vary in thickness, gradually becoming thicker from the neck through the thoracic area to the lumbar area. Sometimes the lowest lumbar disc is slightly thinner than the one above, but this is an exception to the rule.

Each disc (fig. 4) has a soft centre having the consistency of firm jelly (as is found in a packet before the jelly has been diluted with water). The centre is called the nucleus pulposus and it gradually merges with fibres called the annulus fibrosus and these form rings round the nucleus. The annulus has several layers like an onion. They join the vertebra above to the vertebra below. Instead of passing vertically from one to the other these fibres pass obliquely and adjacent layers have opposite oblique fibres. The purpose of this arrangement is that rotation to one side will be limited by one set of fibres and rotation to the other side will be limited by the alternate layer.

Discs are insensitive structures because they have no nerve endings in the

19

nucleus or annulus. The overlying ligaments attached to the annulus, however, have nerve endings and if these ligaments are torn or stretched by disc displacements then pain follows. This explains why, if you have a heavy fall, you may not immediately feel pain even though damage has been done to the inner fibres. Many a person has fallen, say, from a horse, has got up and felt a bit shaken but suffers no pain and he naturally makes the assumption that no damage has been done. Only later does pain occur because swelling of the disc develops during the next few days sufficient to stretch the sensitive adjacent ligaments.

The ligaments outside the annulus fibrosus join the vertebrae together right from the skull to the pelvis. Ligaments not only join the vertebral bodies together but also join the transverse and spinous processes of adjacent vertebrae.

When describing the spine it is useful to look upon two vertebrae and the disc between as a single vertebral segment. The segment includes the ligaments and muscles which join them, the holes between the processes (the foramina) and the central canal through which the spinal cord runs. In front of the spinal canal are the discs and vertebral bodies and behind are the two apophyseal joints. These joints not only help movement between adjacent vertebrae but to some extent they control the type of movements which can occur. Were it not for these joints the vertebral bodies could move in all planes of forward and backward bending, side bending and rotation. Free movement is not feasible in every plane in the normal spine due to the opposing surfaces of these joints. Anyone who is learning to manipulate the spine must understand the ways in which the joints assist or limit movement. Skilled and painless manipulation is only possible when these small joints are taken into consideration during manipulation. This is one explanation why one method of manipulation may be painful and harmful, while another may be painless and beneficial.

The disc acts both as a *cushion* to absorb shocks and as a buffer to keep the vertebrae apart. They are kept apart not merely by the cushion effect but by the distension of the disc by fluid. It is a dynamic mechanism not just a passive hinge. This pressure within the disc is about 100 lb per square inch (7 kg per square centimetre or 690 kPa). The pressure is increased when standing and decreased when lying down. The load-bearing capacity of such a small structure is phenomenal when healthy – professional weight-lifters can lift 374 lb (170 kg) and this is of course added to the existing 7 kg/sq.cm pressure. Furthermore, if a young healthy person suffers a compression injury like falling off a horse on to the base of his spine or falling from a tree on to his feet, it is the bone structure which gives way first rather than the cartilage – and a fracture occurs. This is not so of course if the disc structure is already faulty. In a degenerating disc only minimal pressure is needed to displace it as, for example, picking up a pencil from the floor. Even coughing is enough to displace a fragment of a degenerated disc.

A sponge can absorb water and discs can do the same, but a sponge is passive in the sense of loosing water when squeezed and allowing water to flow in when released. The spongy properties of the cartilage are increased by the additional active absorption of water. If this were not so, weight bearing in the erect position would squash the discs flat whereas healthy discs remain turgid.

The exchange of fluid is gradual. During the day, when weight bearing, we are compressing our discs and slowly we reduce in height by about $\frac{1}{2}$ in (1 cm). During the night, when lying down, pressure is reduced and we regain the height. You can prove this point by having someone measure your height before and after sleep. Measurement differences of up to $\frac{3}{4}$ in (2 cm) have been recorded. Astronauts became taller in space flights by as much as $\frac{3}{4}$ in. Babies' discs are ninety per cent water and this percentage of fluid diminishes with time, but even at seventy years of age the water content of discs is about seventy per cent. Also with the passage of time the fibrous content increases and the elasticity decreases so that most elderly people shrink in height from $\frac{1}{2}$ – 2 in (1 – 5 cm) due to thinning of the discs.

There are twenty-three discs in the spine and they form a quarter of the spinal column. The average length of the spine is $23\frac{1}{2}$ in (60 cm), 6 in (15 cm) of which is made up of cartilage so that the total of 6 in is increased to $6\frac{1}{2}$ in (16 cm) each night and decreased again each day. The fluid in the discs derives from the vertebral bodies above and below and this interchange of fluid is vital for disc health and toughness. If, due to injury, the fluid interchange is impaired then the cartilage begins to degenerate. It loses some of its elasticity and strength. It can swell up or it can fragment.

The fluid interchange between the vertebral bodies and the soft centre of the disc occurs through the cartilage which separates the bone from the nucleus pulposus. This cartilage has numerous perforations which allow plasma from the blood to provide nutrients to keep the cartilage alive. Without this free interchange of fluids and nutrients the cartilage degenerates and disintegrates. Sleep in the horizontal plane, whatever else it does to the body's nervous system, provides an essential period for proper nourishment of the discs. This is why it is sometimes necessary, if you have a disc problem, to stay in bed. The rest facilitates better nutrition for the discs while they are repairing.

The spinal cord is an extension of the brain and runs down the spine within the spinal canal (fig. 3). At all levels nerves are going into and out of the spinal cord and where they emerge from the spine through the foramina they are called nerve roots. The spinal cord is covered by three layers of tissue known as meninges. These highly sensitive layers are separated by fluid for lubrication and free movement of the spinal cord within the spinal canal. It may not be realized that when we flex our necks forward fully, the whole spinal cord moves within the canal and its lowest point may rise as much as 2 in (5 cm). The spinal nerves which emerge from the cord, therefore, have to be very elastic and have to be free to move within the spinal canal. This applies especially to the spinal nerves as they transverse the foramina. Any tethering of the cord or nerves causes tingling or pain when the neck is flexed, or when the limbs are moved.

Within the spinal canal there are numerous blood vessels, both arteries and veins, which run longitudinally and which link several segments of the spine together. This is important because if the spinal cord is deprived of blood even for a short time serious damage follows and the spinal cord cells do not recover once they have ceased to function. There is a contrast here with nerves in the trunk and limbs because such peripheral nerves generally recover even when badly damaged.

2 PATTERNS OF BACK PAIN

Pain in the back shows itself in many different ways. Your own back pain is likely to be similar to that experienced by many other people. The patterns of back pain occur frequently enough to be divided into categories and that is why this chapter is devoted to these varied patterns. In addition, a description of typical patterns will help you to find one which fits in with your own symptoms.

My forty years of practical experience and study of back problems has led me to classify back pain into the syndromes which follow. A *syndrome* is the medical word used to cover a combination of symptoms. This is a convenient term because the precise diagnosis of back pain is not always feasible. Clear-cut patterns of pain and associated signs and symptoms are well recognized. Even though the cause of the syndrome may not be completely understood, the term is useful for descriptive purposes. Just as you can have one type of headache and it can be labelled congestive or migrainous without the precise mechanism of the headache being worked out, so we can have episodic or ligamentous syndromes in the spine without knowing the exact causes of the pain.

A disease of the spine, for example, tuberculosis, expresses itself in a well-known manner and the signs and symptoms are well defined and are described in medical textbooks. The same applies in other diseases, say, rheumatoid arthritis of the cervical joints, or cancer of the spinal bones or transverse myelitis of the spinal cord. These are specific diseases of the spine but they account for less than one per cent of patients suffering back pain. Most of the other ninety-nine per cent of patients have mechanical disorders of the back, if we include degenerative changes in our list of mechanical disorders.

If you think of how a car works then, if something goes wrong with the engine, that is a 'mechanical' fault whereas, if the bodywork starts to wear, that is like a 'degenerative' change. It is similar with the spine. Such conditions make up the vast majority of causes for back pain. It will be some satisfaction for you to learn that this is so and that back pain does not imply serious disease. Furthermore I am sure you will be relieved to know that there are effective methods of treatment for most back pains.

Looking for clues

Some general observations about signs and symptoms will be helpful here before describing the common patterns of back pain.

Mechanical disorders in the spine cause pain related to activity, i.e., the pain does not normally occur at rest. If mechanically-produced pain is severe the pain may continue even at rest but usually the adoption of another position will reduce the severity of that pain.

Mechanically-produced pain is usually intermittent and is accentuated by certain movements or activity. 'Avoiding those movements or activities usually reduces the pain.

'Stretch pain' and 'squeeze pain' have a different significance. For example, if you feel a pain on the right side of your neck while side bending to the left, there is something on the right side of your neck which hurts by stretching. Adhesions and tight joint ligaments cause this type of stretch pain. Where pain occurs on the right side of your neck with side bending to the right it means that compression of some structure or other hurts on the right side. A nerve is being compressed or some structure is getting in the way of the movement – perhaps a narrow foramen or perhaps a disc fragment blocking the movement.

Pain has varying intensity, distribution, periodicity and quality. The severity of pain is difficult to judge because there is nothing to measure it by, nothing to compare it with and even if you say your pain is like toothache this is no guide to its severity because toothache can be mild or intense. One wit said that pain is measured in 'Hells or Decihells'! Some describe a cut finger as agony and excruciating, others as a trifle. The site of the pain will guide you to its origin; most superficially-produced pain is felt accurately but deep sources of pain are poorly localized. Superficial pain is often sharp and intermittent whereas deep pain is dull and continuous. Really severe pain is accompanied by other signs like a raised pulse rate and blood pressure, increased breathing and sweating, sometimes nausea and vomiting (a 'sickening' pain). Persisting severe pain leads to shock with pallor, rapid thin pulse, trembling and cold sensations.

Pain which is intermittent and having its own rhythm unrelated to position or activity is more often than not due to distension of an organ or tube. The only pain in the back, of this type, is kidney pain.

If you feel burning, tingling, cutting, hot, cold or numb sensations these are usually due to irritation of the nerves where the sensation is felt or at some site along the pathway of the nerves which travel to those skin areas. For example, pressure on a nerve in a foramen can cause tingling in the arm and fingers.

Tenderness (which means it hurts to press it) usually implies a local problem though not always so. The skin can be tender, for example, at the site of a boil which inflames the skin, or the local nerves may be irritable as in shingles, or the nerve supply to the skin may be irritated at some distance from the skin and still make the skin tender to pressure.

You will experience *stiffness* as a sensation of restricted movements sometimes associated with pain and sometimes not. When accompanied by pain the pain is usually the cause of the limited movements. Because it hurts to move, the movement is avoided and restriction noticed. If no pain is present then you may be aware of stiffness because previously you were able to move better and more freely. Some people are far more flexible than others and stiffness is an individual characteristic. A lissom person may have average ranges of movement yet feel stiff because they were freer before. Stiffness which develops with rest usually implies a mild degree of inflammation in a joint.

Stiffness is felt in muscles which have been in a slight degree of contraction for a long time. Stiffness is felt in the spine in some back syndromes, say, after sitting or lying. Stiffness which develops during or after activity implies that chemical by-products of muscle contraction are accumulating in these muscles. Stiffness that diminishes with activity implies that such chemical substances had previously accumulated and the activity disperses them. Reduced mobility is called hypomobility.

Mobility If your joints are too mobile we call it hypermobility and many people are hypermobile in all or many joints. Such folk are vulnerable in the sense that, although their joints are not easily sprained, when they are sprained the ligaments repair badly and the joint remains unstable. Excess of mobility can occur in one or two joints of the spine as a compensating mechanism for poor mobility of adjacent joints. A combination of excess and reduced mobility in an area of the spine can be misleading, because the total ranges of movements may be normal. Such combinations of hypermobility and hypomobility are not well recognized even by many doctors or therapists who deal with back problems. Recognition of such cases requires detailed examination to test each inter-vertebral joint and by taking 'mobility' X-rays to compare full forward bending with full backward bending.

Adhesions

What they are Whenever inflammation occurs in the body, whether from infection or mechanical or chemical irritation, some extra fluid is formed at the site of the inflammation and this fluid is sticky. It sticks or adheres one adjacent surface to another and in due course fibrous tissue forms across the surfaces. That is why these tissues are called adhesions. They limit movement between layers which should move freely. After any sprain, for example, a sprained ankle, there is swelling, sticky fluid forms and adhesions occur. It is nature's way of repairing. All well and good if the tissue repairs well and the adhesions disperse, but sometimes the adhesions persist and lead to permanent stiffness in the affected joints.

If you have a simple sprain of the ankle, only one joint is involved. It is impossible to walk normally with a stiff and painful ankle, but by exercises and normal walking the fibrous adhesions gradually stretch and mobility is restored. Such normal mobility, however, would not occur if the joint had been kept still.

Exercise and movements are desirable in the early stages of joint sprains but it becomes even more important to move the joint strongly once repair has taken place. In almost all ankle sprains simple exercises are sufficient to restore full mobility but occasionally the adhesions are tough and will not yield. It then hurts to stretch the adhesions because the fibres pull on the sensitive membranes in the joint. Consequently, if you do not try to stretch the adhesions, permanent restriction of movement can follow. Such adhesions may then have to be stretched strongly by manipulation to restore mobility once more.

Now, if we apply the same principle to the spine, assuming that adhesions have formed round a nerve root or in the capsule of an apophyseal joint and it hurts to stretch, it is natural for most people to avoid the pain and to keep the area stiff. We can manage most daily activity without necessarily moving a sprained spinal joint. It is easy to avoid moving parts of the spine, consequently spinal adhesions are common and occur more frequently than in the joints of the limbs. There is no formal medical term for adhesions in spinal joints but the osteopathic profession (which has made a great study of back problems) has named such spinal joint restrictions as osteopathic lesions.

What to look for   In this syndrome you will feel pain in the centre of the spine or on one side and at any level of the spine from the skull to the pelvis. The pain is accentuated by stretching, i.e., the pain is felt centrally with forward or backward movements. There is no pain at rest unless you adopt a position which involves stretching the painful area. Stiffness is experienced because of pain rather than because of much limitation of movements. In most cases only one joint is affected by adhesions though of course several can be involved. In those cases the restrictions are greater but rarely is there serious limitation of mobility. Occasionally the pain spreads above and below the level of the adhesions or radiates along related nerve pathways to cause referred pain elsewhere. The muscles round the affected point are tense and tender. There may be some disturbances of function in related structures, i.e., in the organs or tissues which have a nerve supply derived from the spinal cord at the same level as the joint in question. For example, you could experience a stomach pain which derives from adhesions in the lower thoracic joints.

As a rule you will have a history of some previous sprain of the spinal joint due to an injury. Another explanation is that repeated movements or postures which put minor strain on the joint over a long period of time have a cumulative effect. In other words several minor stresses can be equivalent to one major sprain. You may have forgotten an original injury because adhesions take time to form and the original incident may not have been severe. It hurt perhaps for a day or two then subsided and the incident is forgotten. Many minor restrictions of mobility are present without causing symptoms. Only when another sprain occurs and the spine is examined for something else are those adhesions discovered.

What can be done   It is probable that the majority of spinal joint sprains recover fully and a complete recovery of normal mobility occurs spontaneously. This is more likely if you engage in exercises which stretch and move the spine normally. Most of us would benefit from some general stretching exercises for the spine as described in chapter five and fewer joint sprains would become chronic. If these minor sprains and adhesions lead to persisting limitations of mobility then the affected joints are not working fully, circulation is impaired

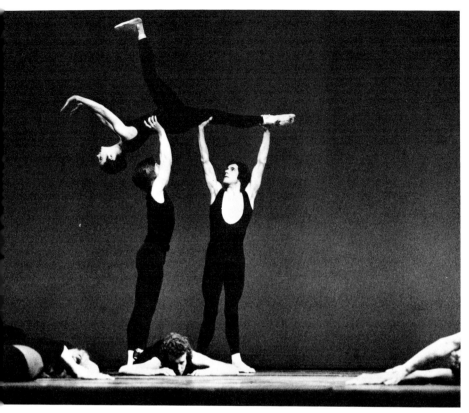

Dancers practise to increase muscle endurance and stamina.

and this leads to degenerative changes later in life with perhaps disc displacements (see page 35). In other words the adhesions syndrome can lead to disc
lesions years later and because of this they are more important than the immediate
symptoms indicate.

If you think that your pain tallies with the above description try stretching
exercises (pages 69–85). If these exercises are insufficient to release the adhesions
then manipulation is the most appropriate form of treatment. Manipulation as a
therapy will be needed because you are not always able to exert enough stretch on
the restricted joint yourself. Manipulation when performed correctly and
skilfully can exert a direct and specific influence on any joint of the spine. The art
of manipulation depends on the ability of the practitioner to combine the forces
he uses such that the maximum leverage occurs precisely at the level of the
restricted joint. Such skill takes a great deal of practice to perfect. Clearly those
engaged in continuous practice are likely to be more skilled than those who
manipulate only on rare occasions. The concert pianist practises his art daily to
maintain a high standard. This applies equally to the art of manipulation.
Examples of manipulation are illustrated on pages 103 and 106.

Strained ligaments

What they are   When a joint is sprained badly and ligaments are torn the repair is sometimes incomplete and the ligaments never regain their original length and strength. This makes the joint feel weak and unstable. If you have a torn ligament you will not have much confidence in the joint because you sense this weakness. This applies to the spine as well as to the joints of the limbs.

Similarly if a joint is stretched to its limit and the stretch is maintained for too long the ligaments then elongate and begin to hurt. If you have ever painted the ceiling you will know what is meant by this (p. 56). The pain is nature's warning that the stretch has gone too far or has been sustained too long.

This type of pain occurs commonly in the lumbar spine or in the neck but not in the thoracic spine. This is because the lumbar area and the neck are more mobile and are subjected to more injury or to more continuous stretch.

What to look for   Early on in this syndrome, you will experience pain after adopting a position of stretch for too long – the commonest example of this is when sitting low in an easy chair without any back support, say, watching television for a couple of hours. At the end of this time there is a vague ache in the centre of the spine low down near the pelvis and the spine feels stiff when rising into a standing position. It may take two or three moments for the ache and stiffness to wear off.

You will probably notice a similar pain and stiffness if you work for hours at a desk, say, with the neck flexed forward. Your neck will then ache. Secretaries and chess players are likely to suffer this type of stiffness!

Most people who experience this pain have it centrally rather than to one side, but if you adopt a position which stretches one side of the spine too much then that side will eventually protest. This sort of back or neck problem is very slow to develop. It may have originated with a severe sprain which has not mended well or has not been allowed to recover because of your work or by the poor posture which you normally adopt.

As the symptoms recur and as the ligaments weaken still more you will be aware that it takes shorter periods of time for the pain and stiffness to start following the adoption of the faulty posture. Eventually the ligaments may become so irritable and weak that pain occurs immediately the strained posture is assumed. At this stage there can be some confusion between ligamentous strain pain and the adhesions syndrome previously described because adhesions also give rise to pain on immediate stretch. However, weak ligaments take a long time to show up whereas injury causes immediate pain. Considering the medical history of the patient helps a doctor or therapist to determine whether he or she has the ligamentous syndrome or the adhesions syndrome.

An examining doctor or therapist who is adept at testing the spine can easily distinguish these two types because the adhesions syndrome causes restriction of mobility and the ligamentous stretch syndrome causes excess of mobility. Furthermore the ligamentous-stretch person has a full range of overall

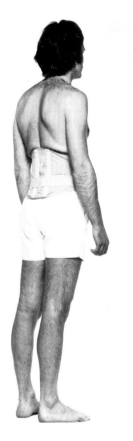

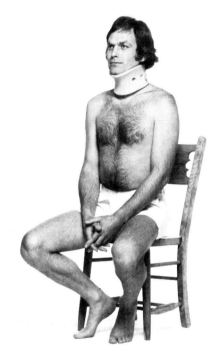

LEFT: A corset prevents too much bending. It can protect the lower back and sacro-iliac joints.

BELOW: A collar prevents movement of an injured neck.

movements and may well be in the 'double-jointed' class of person who is excessively lissom.

Doctors or therapists unfamiliar with this syndrome may examine their patients and when they find that there are no restrictions of spinal movements they tend to dismiss the case as 'functional' or unimportant.

A word of warning. Ligamentous weakness is not easy to treat. Certainly manipulation is no answer. In fact when weak joints are manipulated, especially if treated too forcibly, the joint pain is accentuated. Such inadvisable manipulation has brought discredit on manipulation as a method of treatment and it shows how important it is that the manipulator should be skilled in diagnosis as well as in technique.

What can be done   If you have a ligamentous back pain it may recover quite spontaneously if the affected ligaments are not stretched repeatedly. You may need to alter your standing or sitting or work position to stop the cause of the problem. Such steps need to be taken in any case and some of the symptoms will subside, but despite your best efforts and with the best advice in the world, overstretched ligaments do not always recover their original length and strength.

29

In these cases there is a newish method of injection therapy available and in most cases the ligaments can be artificially strengthened. See page 110 for details of this treatment.

You may find you need support from a corset or neck collar while the ligaments recover. You should also do strengthening exercises to surrounding muscles to provide the support which the ligaments themselves should be giving to the spine. These exercises are designed to increase power in the muscles without stretching the ligaments. We call them isometric exercises (pages 85–91) and they have an opposite purpose to stretching exercises.

Collars and corsets are extensively prescribed by orthopaedic surgeons (pages 29 and 107) and they can be helpful, but to rely solely on external support as the only treatment is, in my opinion, insufficient and incomplete.

More problems arise in the treatment of a spine which has both of the above syndromes, i.e., some joints are too stiff and some joints are too lax. If your back is of this type the weak joints are more likely to cause symptoms than the stiff ones and treatment directed to the ligaments is of primary importance, but manipulating the restricted joints can be helpful and certainly desirable. Even greater skills are required to isolate the restricted joints and to manipulate those only, while at the same time avoiding the risk of over-stretching the weak ligaments.

A curved back   You may also experience ligamentous stretch pain if your back has a structural fault, for example, when the curves of your spine are excessive. An increase of the normal curves is called a kyphosis (round shoulders) in the thoracic area and a lordosis (hollow back) in the cervical and lumbar areas (pages 43 and 47). A lateral curvature is called a scoliosis.

In these cases some of the ligaments are overstretched and elongated whereas other ligaments are understretched and shortened. A good example of this is someone who has one leg shorter than another – a surprising number of people have a leg-length discrepancy. Some years ago I investigated this problem amongst a group of hospital patients and found that twenty-eight per cent had $\frac{1}{4}$ in (7 mm) or more difference in leg length. I compared these figures with those of patients having back pain and found that sixty per cent of back-pain sufferers had $\frac{1}{4}$ in discrepancy or more. The comparison showed that twice as many backache sufferers have unequal leg lengths compared with those without backache. Leg lengths, therefore, can be an important consideration in ligamentous strain.

Both the adhesions syndrome and the ligamentous stretch syndrome may be complicated by an additional factor, namely, a faulty alignment of one vertebra relative to its adjacent vertebra. The bone may be 'out of place'. This is a medically controversial issue but it is fair to say that, although the position of the vertebrae is important, the concept of a spinal lesion (or fault) being just a bone 'out of place' is 'out of date'. The fault is in the joint between the two vertebrae rather than because one vertebra has moved out of alignment with the next

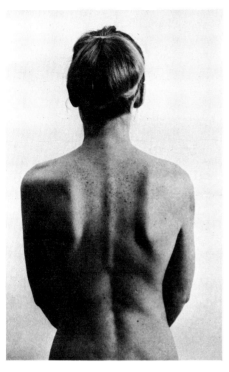

This back, *left*, has a slight kyphosis, lordosis and a gentle curve to the left in the middle of the spine.

vertebra. A full dislocation of a vertebra is possible but it is exceedingly rare and can only be produced by excessive injury sufficient to cause bony damage and even spinal cord damage. **In the two syndromes I have so far described nothing approaching these severe and serious injuries is implied.**

Sudden (or episodic) spinal pain

What it is   According to the dictionary, an episode is a digression, a separate incident in a story to provide variety. If you have an attack of this type of back pain it will certainly be a most unwelcome episode. Most people suffering from this syndrome are completely free from back pain at other times. The attack lasts a few days and is usually over within a week.

What to look for   You may experience the pain in the neck or lumbar region but rarely in the thoracic area. It is characterized by an acute onset for no apparent reason or it follows some trivial action. You may feel something move in the spine. 'It goes out' is an expression often used. The initial pain accompanying the sensation of 'going out' may not itself be severe, but the pain builds up into a crescendo within hours of the onset to such a pitch that it immobilizes you. The event can come on in an awkward place, like in the bathroom, in a car, while out walking with the dog, or even in bed making love. The only advantage in the

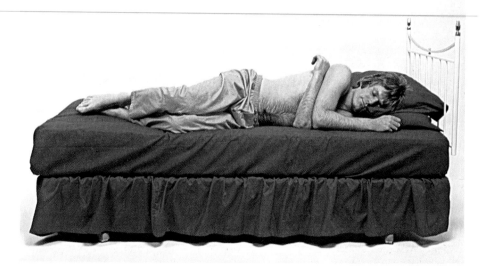

Get up gradually without bending your back. Use your arms to push yourself up sideways.

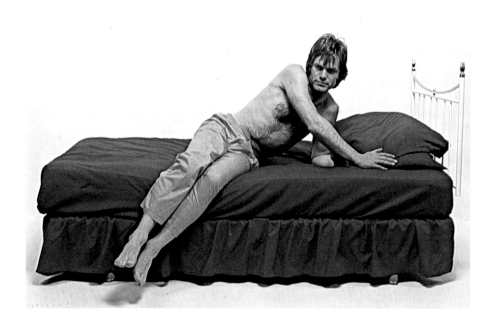

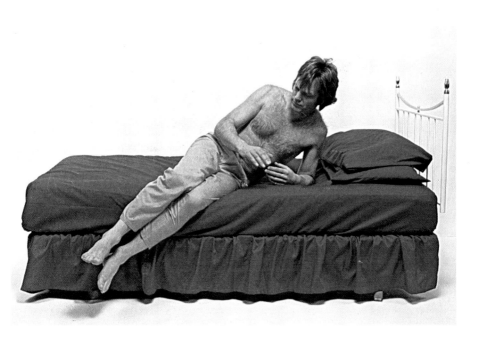

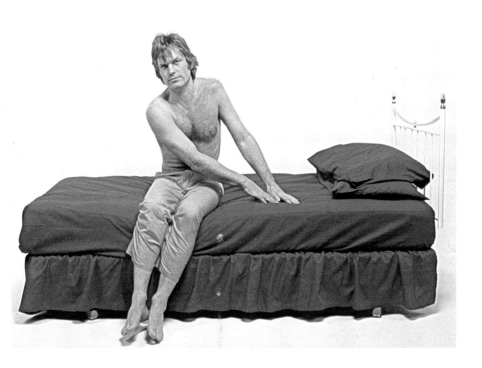

latter situation is that bed is the best place to stay for the next few days!

When horizontal and stationary the pain may subside but the slightest effort to turn over or to get up is excruciating. The pain at first is localized to one site in the spine but soon spreads round the area, right across the lower back or round the ribs or across the shoulders. Any involuntary movement like coughing or sneezing – even deep breathing – exacts its toll of pain and you will try to stay as stationary as possible. Nothing else matters – in fact you can do nothing. The pain is too compelling to think of or do anything but remain stationary. It requires a great effort of will to attempt any alteration of position.

The pain will stay at this intensity for three or four days and then gradually subside; movement becomes feasible again and with it a decrease in the spasm of the muscles round the affected area. As activity returns and you begin to walk about, the pain quickly subsides into a dull ache, but even this disperses in two or three more days. The area may stay stiff a little longer but, unless there are complications, the episode terminates with full restoration of mobility and loss of all pain until the next time.

If you suffer from this type of pain you will soon recognize that you are in this category and will realize also that the two previous syndromes are entirely different from this type. All things have a beginning and the first attack may not be recognized as such by the sufferer. Not knowing what has happened and not realizing its significance you may go on with what you are doing – laying bricks, moving furniture, driving the car, thereby irritating the spine unnecessarily and increasing the severity of the attack unwittingly. Many patients tell me that their first attack was by far the worst because of this.

The usual interval between attacks may last for years, months, or only for weeks and if the common history of such cases is followed the length of the interval shortens, the length of the attack increases and even the quieter recovery phase may persist to give rise to a more continuous dull ache. The next episode could be more severe and change its character – instead of local pain in the spine the pain spreads down the arm or round the chest or abdomen, or into the groin and thigh or into the buttock and calf. About the same time as the pain radiates elsewhere the spinal pain itself usually subsides and the distant pain persists. This radiating pain may continue for weeks or months depending on its cause and degree.

Another feature of an acute episode is spinal distortion. This arises because the pain is less in some positions than others so it is a natural reflex to adopt the position of least pain. The distortion may mean that the pelvis moves sideways and gives rise to a temporary curvature in the spine or the distortion may be backwards to give rise to a temporary kyphosis. In the latter case it becomes impossible to straighten into the erect position. (As the disc displacement is reduced or the swelling subsides these distortions later decrease and usually full normal outward appearances are restored.)

Displaced discs   There are several causes for episodic pain but the majority are caused by disc displacements, commonly known as *slipped discs*. The term 'slipped disc' is misleading because the disc does not slip. Discs when degenerating can swell up, disintegrate and displace. The probable explanation for a typical episodic attack is that the disc swells and the pressure rises so high that something has to give way. It is usually the surrounding and supporting longitudinal ligaments which give way. They tear, they bleed, the chemical substances of tissue damage are liberated and this increases the local swelling, the pain causes reflex muscle guarding to minimize movement, sustained muscle tension then itself causes more pain. If very severe the muscles go into spasm or semi-cramp and everyone knows how painful cramp is.

In simple attacks the swollen disc and torn surrounding ligaments remain thus for a few days, then the swelling diminishes, the disc tensions decrease and the muscle spasm subsides, and the attack is over. What provokes such changes in the discs has so far not been fully worked out, but research workers have found changes in the chemistry of the cartilage and an increase of the lactic acid content of the disc as it swells. We await further studies in the biochemistry of cartilage before we can understand why discs swell and burst. We do know, of course, that increased mechical pressure by lifting, especially when the leverage on the spine is maximized, can increase the risk of disc damage and of acute episodes. But the provocation may be so trivial that the mere increase of pressure at the time is not an adquate explanation for the disc changes. No work and no occupation is free of risk, but certainly manual work, involving excess of lifting or sustained bending, carries a greater risk than office work. Another group of people who are more vulnerable to disc damage are the ones growing up with faulty cartilage – a condition known as osteochondrosis (page 47).

If the swelling is not confined, some of the disc bursts through the surrounding ligaments and the displaced piece presses on the lining membranes (meninges) of the spinal canal and spinal cord. This causes still more pain of a diffuse and ill-defined character. If the pressure increases still more it puts a stretch on a nerve root and then pain radiates in the direction of that nerve root. Finally the pressure can be so great as to compress the spinal cord. This is serious indeed and if a doctor finds his patient so incapacitated he must call in a surgeon to operate and relieve the pressure as quickly as possible. The serious symptoms are loss of sensation in the saddle area of the bottom, loss of control of the bladder or bowel, and loss of sensation of bladder or bowel function.

If a piece of the nucleus of the disc displaces to lie free of the annulus then the adjacent margins of the annulus can join together and healing with fibrous tissue can take place. If you are suffering from this type of trouble you will find that the pain from the stretched annular fibres subsides and the spinal pain disappears. Only the radiating pain persists. After a time – lasting weeks or months – this displaced fragment is absorbed and gets smaller. This is the rule rather than the exception. Thus the majority of sciaticas or brachial neuralgias recover whether treatment is given or not.

Because of the spontaneous natural recovery of most disc displacements it is rarely necessary for a surgeon to be called in. It is estimated that only one person in a thousand back sufferers will ever need surgery. One investigation found that nearly three per cent of the population sought advice about their back problem from their doctor. Of these one in four hundred had to attend hospital and an even smaller proportion had to be operated upon.

Even the worst afflicted can take heart from these figures but when surgery is indicated it must not be unduly delayed. The serious reasons for surgery with disc displacements are as follows:

1. When the pain is too severe to tolerate and there is no other way to reduce the pain to tolerable levels.

2. When the pain is prolonged and incapacity is severe.

3. When the attacks are repeated frequently enough to interfere with the individual's livelihood.

4. When paralysis of muscles develops.

5. When the saddle area is numb and the bowel or bladder function is disturbed.

Nothing of a medical nature is precise and predictable, so that, though the above description of an episodic syndrome is the most typical, there are variations on the theme and there are other causes of acute spinal pain than disc protrusions.

Injury   Acute pain can be due to severe injury and any of the sensitive structures will hurt where damaged – the skin, the ligaments, the muscles, the bones, the meninges and the nerves. You will know that you have damaged yourself because pain is instantaneous following the injury, and quite different from the acute onset of a disc lesion which occurs without obvious provocation (page 33).

Twisting strains   Fairly severe spinal pain can arise from a twisting strain which locks the apophyseal joints – rather like a drawer can be jammed slightly askew in its grooves, so can the facets be caught in an acute angle. This type of sharp spinal pain can be dramatically cured with manipulation. It is relatively uncommon and less painful than a disc protrusion. You will find that some movements are blocked. Such locked joints cannot possibly occur while just bending down, say, to tie up a shoe lace as can happen with a disc protrusion. Although rare, these displacements can occur in the neck, in the lumbar spine and in the sacro-iliac joints (the two joints of the pelvis). There is always an element of twist in the preceding strain.

Inflammation   Apart from the disc protrusions which occur in the neck there is an acute type of neck pain which is inflammatory in origin. It is slower in onset and you may first feel it early in the morning. It can become extremely painful. The pain continues even at rest; if you experience pain when resting this is a sign that your neck is inflamed and the site of that inflammation is in the small apophyseal joints. Quite often only one joint is involved. Sometimes such an attack is a prelude to osteo-arthritis in those joints.

Still another type of acute spinal pain can occur in shingles. This can be confusing because the shingles pain starts three or four days before the typical rash occurs. Yet another acute pain can be a manifestation of gout but as a rule other joints besides the spine help with the latter diagnosis. Some other severe back pains are due to disease. The onset is gradual and the pain is unrelated to activity or rest.

What can be done for acute episodic pain? It all depends upon the stage at which the condition has arrived. In some people who have previous experience it is possible to do something effective in the first few hours of the attack and when successful the attack can be reduced from a week to one day. This can only occur if the disc is merely bulging and not fully displaced. Then a strong pulling (traction) technique (page 108) can reduce the bulge. In a locked joint a twisting manipulation (page 105) can release the locking and give relief.

If a competent manipulator is not available (and he must be a competent diagnostician too) then what can you do? The safest 'do it yourself' manipulation is to stretch your own spine by hanging from a bar or bannister and allow the weight of the two legs to exert a traction force on the spine. Even if this does no good it cannot do any harm and is worth trying. The way to do it is to find a hold for your hands, ideally within easy reach when standing. The most readily available place is a door – opened, of course. Cling to the top of the door near the hinges to make sure you do not pull the door down! A cloth or a newspaper will make the grip on top of the door more comfortable for the hands.

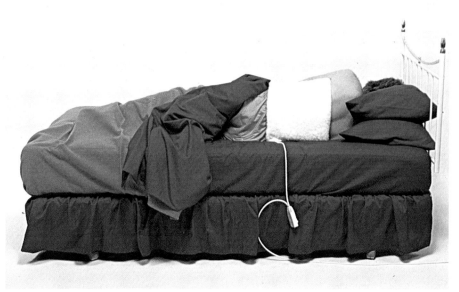

An electric pad gives local heat to the affected part of the back.

Then slowly bend at your knees leaving your toes on the floor, relaxing the legs all the while to help the stretching of the spine. It is no use bracing your arms as if for a chin-up exercise, because all the muscles will contract. By this method you attempt to relax all the muscles of the body except the hands. The legs act as a dead weight to pull the vertebrae apart. It is not an easy thing to do and if you are unable to relax the legs well it will be unsuccessful. No harm, however, will be done by the attempt. While hanging there, and having relaxed fully for a while, try tilting the pelvis to and fro especially to arch the spine backwards. You cannot over-stretch the spine in this way because your hands will tire long before you overdo it. As you retake the pressure on your feet do it gradually so that the disc is not suddenly compressed again, otherwise you just give yourself another unpleasant twinge.

The other important step is to lie down and take the weight off the spine. If you have had a previous attack you will recognize the early warning 'gone out' sensation with moderate pain. Do not provoke the attack into more severity by continuing your gardening or washing, for instance. Lie down as soon as you can and apply heat. Heat is a comfort because it helps to reduce muscular tension. If the muscles are in spasm the heat will make very little difference and then drugs may be necessary. A hot-water bottle is the most usually available form of heat but it is not necessarily best. Preferably use a miniature electric blanket or electric pad (page 39) which maintains its temperature at a constant level. Have it as hot as you can bear it but avoid burning the skin. A hot bath is not recommended because it can be a struggle to get in and out of the bath and there is a risk of bending forwards with the knees straight – just the very thing which 'put the back out' in the first place. A shower solves the problem of washing without bending.

As the pain subsides try gentle movements in bed, lying on your back and arching up and down slowly or reaching down first with one leg and then the other (page 35). Gentle intermittent movements help the circulation and the alternating relaxation and contraction of the muscles reduces the accumulation of chemical by-products in the muscles. Do not, of course, continue any exercise or movement which provokes more muscle spasm.

It is not necessary to stay lying on your back. If you can turn on to one side or even lie prone (face downwards) it sometimes give more relief than the supine position. When attempting to rise up from the horizontal position (as will be necessary to pass water), turn on to one side first, put your feet over the side of the bed and then push yourself up all in one piece (pages 36–7). Have a commode near the bed if possible. A bed pan is more awkward and requires athletic capabilities! Although rising from bed can be extremely painful, no serious harm can come from the struggle so long as it is done slowly, deliberately and without jerking.

Mercifully the pain diminishes in a few days, and then the more the muscles are used the better so long as the activity does not increase the pain. The earliest exercises should be done horizontally as already suggested. Then in a sitting or standing position try side bending several times (pages 76–7). Avoid forward bending until much later. Most disc protrusions occur in forward bending and

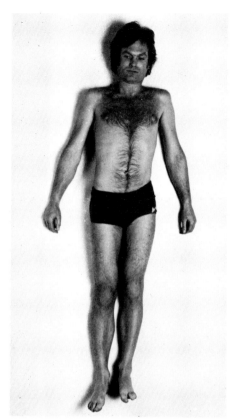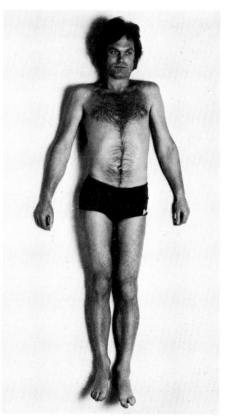

This gentle exercise involves reaching down first with the right leg ... followed by reaching down with the left leg. Continue alternating like this.

there is no point in risking more trouble. Side bending is safe and backward bending can be managed in most cases without risk of pain.

If the episode proceeds to a full disc protrusion then the problem becomes quite different. No longer can one expect a reduction of the displacement because the piece which has come out of position is larger than the space or channel from which it came; the only hope is to alter the relationship of the protrusion and the nerve roots. It is sometimes, though not always possible, to achieve this by manipulation but again you must be in expert hands. Any injudicious or unskilled manipulation could accentuate the problem rather than relieve it. Such precautions need to be even more carefully taken if the disc protrusion has caused some loss of conduction in the nerve root resulting in numbness or loss of power.

During the recovery phase it is necessary to be cautious because, even though pain has subsided, the healing process is not yet complete. It is estimated that even with full restoration of normal position within the disc and adjacent joints it takes about six weeks for repair to be strong. If you have suffered an acute episode you are well advised to avoid provoking the spine during these six weeks. A second attack during the healing phase takes even longer to repair.

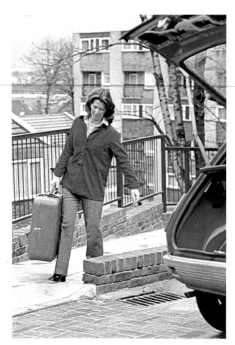

Carrying a heavy suitcase in one hand is hard work for your back. It only makes matters worse to bend as you lift it into the car.

Two suitcases are better than one! The weight becomes evenly distributed. Bend your knees rather than your back.

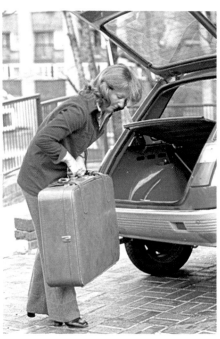

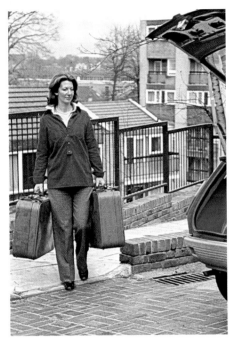
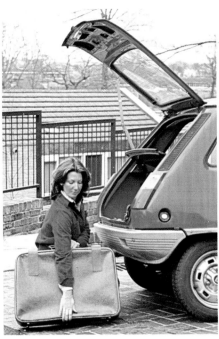
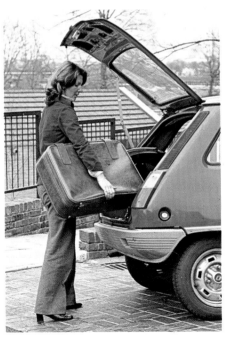
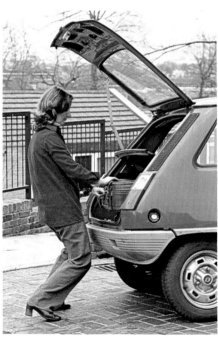

Chronic back pain

Spondylosis and osteo-arthritis   When disc protrusions recur they may lead on to more persisting and chronic pain. This is a feature of unresolved disc protrusions. Chronic degenerative changes lead on to spondylosis. Then X-rays show thinning of the disc spaces, thickening of the margins of the vertebrae and hardening of the adjacent bony surfaces. All of these changes can lead to persisting back and neck pains, and the outlook is discouraging but some light is visible on the horizon because it is an observed fact that there are fewer severe disc displacements in the elderly compared with the thirty to fifty age group and it is rare indeed for recurring episodic attacks of pain and subsequent spondylosis to go on to osteo-arthritis.

Here I would like to make a distinction between spondylosis and osteo-arthritis of the small spinal joints (apophyseal joints). This distinction is very definite though even in medical literature the two conditions are confused. The reasons for the confusion are that both are degenerative in nature, both show bony spurs (or osteophytes) and in many people signs of both conditions are present. Just because there are some overlapping features, however, it is not necessary to confuse these two conditions. Furthermore it is important for you to know which of them you suffer from because with spondylosis the prognosis is better than with osteo-arthritis. With spondylosis there is a good chance of spontaneous recovery and much less pain as age advances, whereas with osteo-arthritis the prospects are poor in many instances and the condition tends to increase with age.

How to tell the difference between spondylosis and osteo-arthritis

1. Spondylosis affects the vertebral bodies and the discs whereas osteo-arthritis affects only the small apophyseal joints.

2. Spondylosis is not primarily inflammatory though some inflammation may follow, whereas osteo-arthritis is essentially inflammatory.

3. Spondylosis affects different levels of the spine from osteo-arthritis. Spondylosis is most common in the lower neck, the mid-thoracic area and the lower lumbar joints. Osteo-arthritis only affects the upper cervical and the lowest two lumbar joints.

4. Spondylosis leads to intermittent pain whereas osteo-arthritis is more continuous though punctuated by bad and good phases. With spondylosis it is usually possible to adopt some position of comfort whereas this is less likely with osteo-arthritis. Rest relieves the acute phase of spondylosis. Rest in osteo-arthritis may give marginal relief but being stationary increases the stiffness. Relief is often obtained by continued mild activity.

5. Spondylosis affects the thirty to fifty age group; osteo-arthritis is more likely after sixty years of age.

With any persistent and recurring back pain both spondylosis and osteo-arthritis are possible but those features mentioned above will help you to put yourself into the appropriate category. Sometimes, especially if both conditions co-exist, it is necessary to take X-rays to show where the bony changes have taken place.

What can be done   Spondylosis and osteo-arthritis respond differently to treatment.

Spondylosis needs mobilizing manipulation – the osteopath calls this articulatory manipulation and the physiotherapist calls it Maitland techniques. These techniques are repetitive passive movements to encourage better mobility without harsh or forcible manipulation. They are further designed to increase blood circulation to the affected joints.

Osteo-arthritis on the other hand is better managed by manipulations which incorporate traction to separate the inflamed surfaces. These traction techniques should be done in an intermittent or rhythmic manner and not in a sustained manner. Any strong manipulation which forces the surfaces together merely accentuates the pain and increases the inflammation. Anti-inflammatory drugs can only give temporary relief and their benefit is lost on spondylosis. There is little point in treating a mechanical problem by chemical means. Similarly support in the form of a collar or corset can be of some value in the acute phases of either spondylosis or osteo-arthritis but to continue using such protection tends merely to accentuate the stiffness – especially in osteo-arthritis.

Hollow back

What it is   Lordosis or a hollow back (page 31) can affect the neck or lumbar spine but when it affects the neck it is always secondary to a prominent round back in the thoracic area. If you have a round back your neck is carried forward and your head is forced back because you need to hold it in a comfortable horizontal position to see well and normally. Such a thoracic kyphosis tends also to accentuate the forward curve of the lumbar spine to produce a hollow back.

A lordosis may be present for many years without causing any symptoms whatever but as time goes on and as the discs become narrower (we all grow shorter as age advances), there is less room for the nerves as they emerge from the narrowed intervertebral foramina.

As the back of the vertebrae come closer together more weight is carried at the back of these vertebrae and a number of effects can follow. The spinous processes come into contact with each other. We call this 'kissing spines' and the friction causes local pain and tenderness. The articular process of the vertebra above can drive a wedge into the vertebral arch below, sufficient sometimes to lead to bony damage (spondylolysis) and if it becomes worse there may be a separation and a forward shift of the vertebra above on the one below (spondylolithesis).

What to look for   The overlapping of the apophyseal joints can lead into osteo-arthritis of those joints. Most of these conditions can be diagnosed by X-rays taken on the side, on the front and halfway between. The characteristic pain from your point of view is that backward bending increases the pain whereas other movements, forward and sideways, give relief. You will probably be more comfortable sitting than standing, and prefer to lie on your back than on your front.

What can be done   If you have a hollow back you will find that you experience pain quite differently from most other back sufferers who feel pain when bending forward. Advice on coping with this problem differs, therefore, from the others – low easy chairs and soft beds are advisable. Most people in the other syndromes do better on firm beds (page 96) and sitting upright. The type of manipulation which is appropriate for this condition also differs and involves more forward bending. If forward bending is not included there may be an accentuation of pain. Some of the most severe examples of lordosis (spondylolysis, spondylolithesis and osteo-arthritis) are certainly made worse by forcible manipulation. People suffering from these conditions need protection with corsets and advice on posture. Exercises to correct the hollow back are needed and will be described later (see page 91).

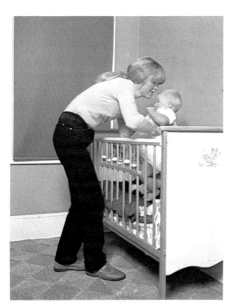 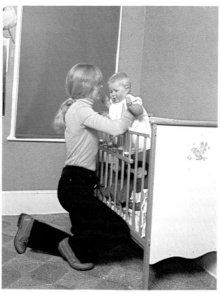

When lifting a baby take care to bend at your knees rather than bending your back – and so avoid unnecessary strain.

A rocking chair is very good for the spine as it provides full support and the rocking movement encourages circulation in the spine.

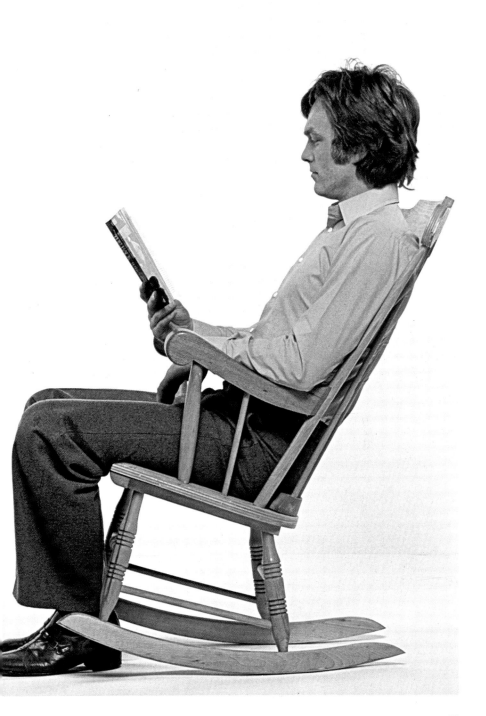

Sacro-iliac syndrome

What it is   The pain is always felt over the sacro-iliac joints (fig. 5). These are located low down in the back where, in most people, there is a dimple. If there is no dimple the position of these joints is found about 4 in (10 cm) above the natal cleft (the groove where the two buttocks meet) and about 2 in (5 cm) on each side of the mid-line.

While it is true to say that pain from the sacro-iliac joint is always felt over the joint, it is far from true to say that all pain in this region must come from the sacro-iliac joints. In fact I would say that more sacro-iliac-area pain derives from the lumbar joints than from the sacro-iliac joints themselves. The pain may radiate into the thigh or into the groin.

What to look for   The commonest cause of sacro-iliac strain is childbirth. The reason for this is that nature arranges to increase the elasticity of the sacro-iliac ligaments to facilitate the birth. It is indeed a marvellous provision of nature, but if the baby is large or the birth is difficult for other reasons the strain on the sacro-iliac ligaments is more than they can take, the ligaments elongate and remain weak. This extra elasticity of sacro-iliac ligaments persists for several weeks and in normal conditions the ligaments regain their previous length and strength and any backache from this cause subsides.

If the ligaments remain long, however, they are relatively easily strained. Lifting the baby, changing nappies, feeding the baby in poor postures (especially if there is a twisting component in these actions) leads to more sacro-iliac strain. The pain is almost always on one side only and may spread into the thigh or groin. If the pain is bilateral, i.e., felt over both sacro-iliac joints it is still possible for the pain to be due to weak ligaments, but bilateral pain is more likely to derive from some inflammation in the sacro-iliac joints or the lumbar spine. When inflammation is present the pain will be more continuous and not influenced by change of position or posture.

Golf is more likely to give rise to sacro-iliac strain than other sports because of the fixation of the hip joints and the twisting of the sacrum during the swing. Any loss of muscle control on swinging beyond the maximum point of control strains the ligaments. You will feel pain at the time of the swing. The pain can increase but will rarely be as severe and crippling as that produced by a disc protrusion.

Manipulation is yet another cause of sacro-iliac strain, especially if repeatedly and forcibly performed in the torsion position (a twisting manipulation). An osteopath may well fall into a trap of his own making here, because the manipulation can initially give relief but because of poor tone in the ligaments they are easily strained again, the patient returns for more manipulation, relief is given but lasts for a shorter time and both patient and manipulator become disheartened. What is really needed then is support in the form of a sacro-iliac binder or corset with a reinforcing band round the pelvis. Sometimes sclerosing injections are necessary to restore tone to the sacro-iliac ligaments (page 110).

The tail bone or coccyx, which is the small bone at the very tip of the spine, is sometimes painful and sitting is uncomfortable. This may be due to an injury or strain at childbirth. It may not have a local origin and, if so, it is a referred pain from above. Lumbar disc lesions are sometimes experienced as pain over and at the tip of the coccyx. After injury adhesions can form in the sacro-coccyxeal joint sufficient to restrict movement and the bone may be displaced. In either case manipulation is effective. This is best achieved by the manipulator using one finger in the rectum and the thumb outside. Good leverage is obtained in this way.

Round back

What it is   A kyphosis or round back (page 31) is an increase in the backward curve of the spine. It is limited to the thoracic area of the spine. The expressions a 'hunch' back, a 'round' back, 'round shouldered' describe this condition. The Hunchback of Notre Dame probably had had tuberculosis of the spine and this disease was common enough early this century but modern hygienic measures with milk and new forms of treatment have taken away the risk of tuberculosis. One of the criticisms levelled against early osteopaths by the medical profession was that they ran a risk of manipulating and making a tuberculous spine worse. Valid as this was, the antagonists of osteopathy overplayed this risk and, in any case nowadays, the risk is exceedingly small.

The commonest present-day cause for a kyphosis is Scheuermann's disease. This used to be known as adolescent kyphosis or osteochondritis; nowadays, osteochondrosis is the name accepted internationally for this condition. The cause is unknown but heredity plays its part. What happens is that the vertebrae, as they are growing, do not grow symmetrically but become wedge shaped. When well marked this distortion of vertebral shapes becomes visible as a group of prominent vertebrae with or without a curvature laterally. During normal growth bone develops from cartilage but in osteochondrosis the growth of the vertebrae is delayed and the conversion of cartilage to bone is faulty. This leads to an area of stiffness, altered shape and sometimes backache.

I have personally done some research into the frequency of osteochondrosis in the population at large and compared this with the frequency of osteochondrosis in patients who have backache. In my series of 925 patients with back pain and 853 individuals whose spines were X-rayed for research purposes I found that 13.1 per cent of the normal population had X-ray signs of osteochondrosis and 42.6 per cent of the back-pain patients had X-ray signs of osteochondrosis. This shows that the condition is fairly common, but also that, in patients who complain of back pain from any cause whatever, three times as many of them have osteochondrosis compared with the population at large.

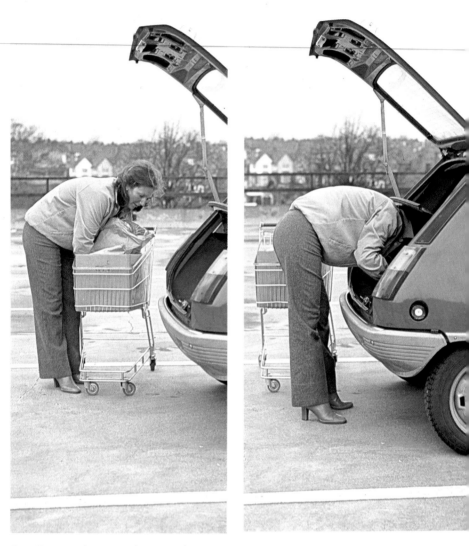

Bending over heavy packages and
attempting to get them into the back of
the car can hurt your back ... but keeping
a straight back and bending at the knees
is much less risky.

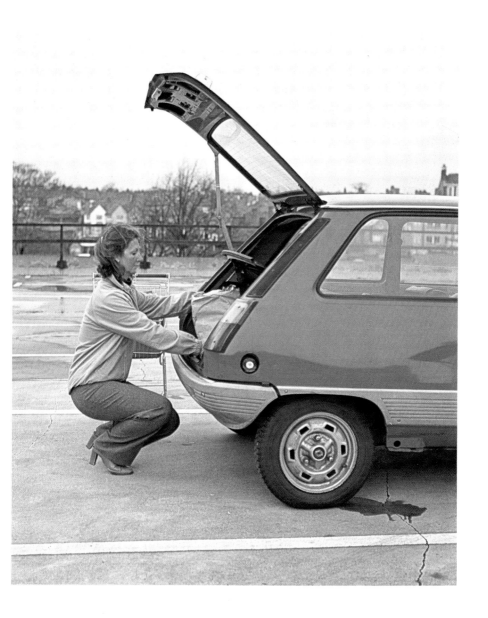

There are other causes of kyphosis in older people and all of us get a bit round as age advances, but a marked kyphosis not previously present and causing pain almost always means some disease is present.

What to look for   If you have osteochondrosis you will have vague backache accentuated by physical effort and lifting strains. There may be pain and signs of disc protrusions either in the thoracic or lumbar areas.

Growing children should be watched for this condition and parents who notice the poor posture of their teenage children should seek advice, especially if the youth complains of backache.

Gentle manipulation is appropriate in osteochondrosis and often effective. Jarring sports like squash and rugby football should be discouraged although swimming, running and athletics (other than jumping) should be encouraged.

What can be done   There are, of course, risks in manipulation, not only when a wrong diagnosis is made, but when giving manipulation at the wrong time in a condition for which it might be appropriate later on. Some manipulations are suitable in a given condition and other types are inappropriate or harmful. But because manipulation occasionally does harm this does not justify the wholesale condemnation of the method in all cases – yet there are some doctors who still adopt this attitude. Likewise, just because an occasional patient dies under, or following, an operation does not justify the condemnation of all surgical procedures.

Soft tissue pain

The soft tissues (as distinct from the hard tissues) are the ligaments, the muscles, the fat and the fascia. The fascia is a sheet of connective tissue separating one layer of muscle from another or separating a layer of muscle from fatty tissue. Ligament pain problems have been described earlier (pages 28–30).

Fatty lumps   Sometimes people develop fatty lumps in the spine especially over the pelvis and buttocks. Occasionally these are painful, but always the pain is superficial and there is tenderness at the site of the nodule when it is squeezed. If a nodule is only tender when pressed against the bone then the tenderness probably arises from some other structure. If a nodule is tender when squeezed then it can be treated by hand massage or by injecting a local anaesthetic and squeezing it vigorously. This breaks up the fat and then it disperses.

Sometimes the fatty tissue is widespread and tender diffusely. This is called panniculitis – the fatty tissue is tender because of the poor circulation flowing through it and the person is usually obese. The best thing to do is to lose some weight and receive strong deep massage.

Muscle pain arises in several ways by tears, by sustained contractions, by unaccustomed physical exertion and by cramp.

A tear in a muscle anywhere in the body is due to violent effort and the pain is instantaneous and severe like a knife being stuck into the muscle. The fibres separate and bunch up. They remain irritable and painful when contracted again. A tear is a rare event in spinal muscles. Most acute spinal pain which is instantaneous comes from ruptured discs or sprained ligaments.

The other acute muscular pain is *cramp*. Most people have experienced cramp, say, in a calf muscle. The pain is severe immediately and the muscle can be both seen and felt to contract violently. No one suffering cramp can be unaware of it. The immediate impulse is to stretch the muscle affected and as a rule this relieves the cramp. Then the pain subsides as quickly as it started. Cramp in the spinal muscles is also rare though I have seen it in gouty patients.

Muscular pain which is gradual in onset is either due to sustained contractions, or related to unaccustomed exertion, or due to 'fibrositis'. An explanation here is helpful. If you contract your shoulder muscles in a sustained way, say, by lifting the arm up and keeping it horizontal you will develop discomfort in the shoulder within two or three minutes. Within five minutes the pain is bad enough to make you want to drop the arm to the side again. The duration of this sustained muscular effort can be lengthened by practice – traffic police and ballet dancers (page 27) can certainly sustain the effort longer than an untrained person – but even for them there is a limit.

The explanation is that during contraction of muscle a chemical change takes place in the fibres and during relaxation the chemistry is restored ready for the next contraction. In this way the alternating contraction and relaxation can be repeated for hours on end without discomfort. During sustained contraction without relaxation, however, the blood flow through the muscles is impeded and the carbon dioxide and other acids accumulate. When concentrated enough these chemical by-products cause pain – telling you to relax.

Another way for muscles to hurt is after unaccustomed exertion. Those stiff aching muscles which you feel on the day following your first game of tennis in the spring are due to accumulation of these by-products. Further on in the season your circulation to the muscles improves and it can cope with the extra chemical changes occasioned by the extra muscular effort.

Yet another form of muscular pain occurs in people with impaired circulation. This is called claudication. Thickening of the arteries leads to poor circulation. Insufficient oxygen reaches the muscles and the accumulated by-products cause pain even with ordinary exercise.

Finally there is muscular pain known as *'fibrositis'*, often brought on by chill. 'Fibrositis' is a misnomer because no inflammation can be detected in these painful sites. The probable explanation is that muscle fibres tighten up selectively and locally and the tension is maintained long enough for muscle by-products to accumulate. These act as further irritants and the situation becomes self-perpetuating. Sometimes the pain will go away and recur when you least expect it. One way of treating these fibrositic areas is to inject the tight fibres with a local anaesthetic and this has the effect of relaxing the muscles and enabling the by-products to disperse. Sometimes the fibrositis is secondary to spinal damage and

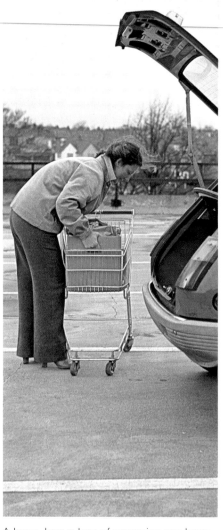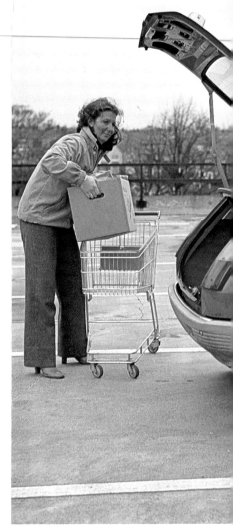

A large, heavy box of groceries can have a disastrous effect on your back ... as you heave it out of the trolley.

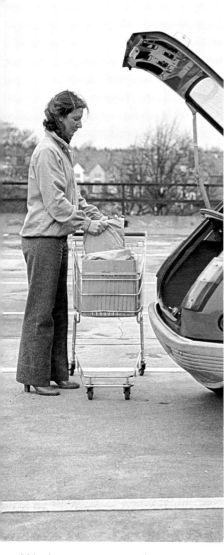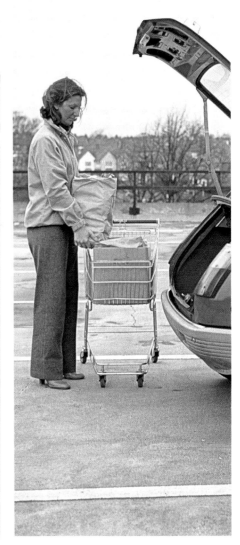

would be better to separate the
groceries into smaller packages ... and
them out carefully one at a time.

this should be corrected first, but despite correct diagnosis and treatment there are some cases of persisting 'fibrositis' which cannot be explained on the basis of mechanical faults. There may well be a biochemical cause for such 'muscular rheumatism'. Deep massage of 'fibrositis' is temporarily effective; so is the rubbing in of liniments but unless the cause of the 'fibrositis' is treated there will be no lasting benefit.

There is a well-recognized syndrome called polymyalgia rheumatica in which the patient (usually elderly) suffers persistent muscular pain especially in the neck and shoulders. This condition does not respond to heat and massage – rather, it is made worse and made more painful with such treatment. Polymyalgia rheumatica is now recognized as one of the stress disorders. An associated arteritis goes with the widespread muscular pain (not to be confused with arthritis). Arteritis is an inflammation of the arteries and if the arteries involved include the eye vessels there is serious risk of permanent visual damage unless correctly treated.

Curvatures of the spine

Curvatures of the spine or scoliosis (page 30) rarely cause pain, and minor ones are often not noticed, but when pronounced they cause distress mainly from the deformity angle rather than from the disability that they cause. I have already mentioned osteochondrosis (page 47) as one cause of a curvature, but these are slight cases. Severe curvatures which are very obvious are usually due to congenital faults but in some cases the cause is unknown.

If you have such a curved spine try strengthening exercises for the spinal muscles (pages 85–91) to reduce the stress on the curves. It's fair to tell you, however, that any reduction of the curvature is unlikely short of drastic surgery. Even surgery should be avoided except in the most serious cases. The psychological and physical damage from the surgery often outweighs the structural benefits.

Neck and shoulder pains

Whiplash injuries As described earlier the neck can be involved in the previous patterns of pain; although ligamentous strain is less likely than in the lumbar spine, whiplash injuries (sustained in car crashes) are common and, in these, an excessive stretch is put on the ligaments which hold the cervical vertebrae together. If you have had a car crash you may notice immediate pain in the neck. Within hours the neck stiffens up due to pain and swelling. The pain is local at first and in most cases the joint involved is between the fifth and sixth cervical vertebrae, but the fourth-fifth cervical level or the sixth-seventh level may be involved as well. Later the pain may radiate to the arms. X-rays taken in the standard manner rarely show any bony damage. X-rays to show full forward bending and full backward bending should be taken to see if any excess mobility occurs at any level. If such excess mobility does show this proves that ligaments have been damaged and torn at the time of the injury.

When a whiplash injury has occurred, especially if mobility X-rays show excess movement, the neck should be splinted with a collar until the ligaments have had time to repair (page 109). In severe cases repair takes as long as six weeks.

The adhesions syndrome is common in the neck and can affect any level. When upper cervical joints are involved the pain may well radiate upwards into the head. Headaches are a frequent sequel to the upper cervical joint strains and to adhesions. You will usually experience this type of headache at the back of the head.

Manipulation is very effective in the adhesions syndrome. Skilful, accurate manipulation at the level of the restricted joint is essential. Excessive force or faulty localization of manipulation can do more harm than good.

Acute episodes of neck pain can affect the lower cervical joints. The acute 'wry' neck is usually due to a disc protrusion which should be reduced by the appropriate manipulation and traction. Disc lesions and apophyseal joint strain can cause pain in the arm extending down to the hand. Tingling or numbness may ensue and occasionally weakness of muscles follows.

A collar is useful for an acute pain in the neck, but the continued use of collars after six weeks of symptoms is inadvisable because adhesions may develop and persist.

Chronic pain   Spondylosis and osteo-arthritis of the apophyseal joints are both degenerative in nature and the differences between the two conditions were discussed on page 42. Most of what was said there applies to the neck as well as to the lumbar spine.

Headaches   Upper cervical joint lesions can cause headaches, 'fibrositis', giddiness and occasionally disturbed vision and hearing. *Migraine* is not primarily due to mechanical lesions in the neck, but such faults can cause an increase in frequency and severity of the migrainous attacks. If you suffer from migraine you ought to have the neck examined and any lesions there treated by manipulation.

After concussion, headaches are common and may be due to temporary brain damage, but if headaches persist then the neck joints should be examined lest lesions there are perpetuating the headaches.

Nervous-tension headaches are expressed by muscular tension at the base of the skull and they can be relieved by local massage, relaxation and manipulation, but the underlying causes of the nervous tension must also be dealt with.

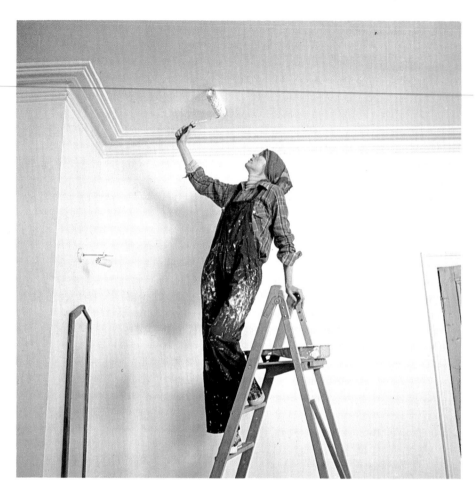

There is no way of avoiding neck ache when painting a ceiling. Just stop every now and again and don't go on for too long.

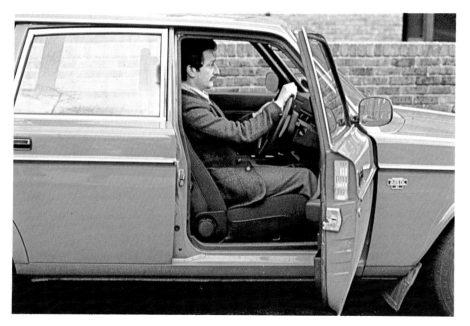

A car seat which provides neck and back support, like this one supplied by Volvo, is both safe and comfortable.

Psychological back pain

In back pain caused by psychological factors little or no local cause can be found for the pain. An underlying depression or anxiety state may manifest itself in the spine and the area of that pain may be influenced by some minor mechanical problem in the spine. The pain tends to be more persistent and constant than a simple mechanically-produced pain. This type of pain is rarely relieved by ordinary pain-relieving drugs. The symptoms are accentuated in times of stress whether this is mental or emotional or even physical and when there is pressure of work or greater responsibility.

'Oh! He is a pain in the neck,' 'She gets my back up' are phrases in the English language which illustrate the influence of tension. In this case the tension is created by some irritating other person. What actually happens is that the irritating person makes you tighten up muscularly. If the muscular tension is maintained long enough this causes physical pain in the muscles.

Our whole lives are influenced by mental, emotional and physical factors interplaying with each other. The spine is the telephone exchange between the body and the brain. Mental strain distorts the emotions and causes physical pain. Emotional distress causes mental tensions and impairs physical performance. Physical pain leads to mental anxiety and aggravates emotional imbalance. All of these influences may be at work, leading to or resulting from spinal pain, so that every individual who suffers spinal pain of a physical nature will develop a mental or an emotional response. In the same way mental and emotional conflicts can express themselves forcibly in back problems.

3 WHAT THE DOCTOR OR THERAPIST IS LOOKING FOR

History   When patients complain of back pain the routine medical procedure is to take a history. The doctor or therapist will want to know when the pain started, how it began, where it was located, how severe it was, whether the pain spread and where it spread to, and how the symptoms have changed since the onset. He will want to know about pins and needles, numbness and if weakness or stiffness have developed and when. A clear history is of great help to the doctor or therapist and the time sequence helps to differentiate one syndrome from another. The past medical history is important too, whether there have been accidents, illness, operations, injuries at sport, falls on to the spine. The patient's occupation with its strains and stresses on the spine may be significant. In women the number of pregnancies, normal or abnormal births, and any back pain experienced at these times will also be important. Finally the patient's general health is relevant to any spinal problem.

Examination   When examining the spine the doctor or therapist notes the posture, body outline, spinal contours, pelvic symmetry, leg lengths, the inclination of the head and neck and shoulder levels. These observations are repeated when seated and lying down. During the change of position the doctor notices whether difficulty is experienced when moving into those positions.

Throughout the history-taking and examination, the doctor is making a note of the demeanour of the patient, trying all the while to assess the type of individual he is dealing with. The responses of patients to questions and tests give a great deal of information about the character and psychology of the patient. A physician is on the look-out for the patient who exaggerates or minimizes the symptoms. He is looking at the patient as a whole human being not just looking at a faulty joint. The patient is a whole person with a back problem – not a back problem in isolation.

Detailed examination of the spine should include palpation of the area of pain, testing for the distribution of pain and for movements in each area of the affected joints, assessing muscular tension round the affected joints, locating tender sites in muscles or over ligaments.

X-rays   If the history and the physical examinations do not enable the doctor to determine the syndrome from which the patient is suffering, extra help can be obtained by taking X-rays of the spine. Here I would like to stress the importance of *functional* X-rays. By this I mean X-rays which give additional information about weight bearing and ranges of movement.

Patients often say that they have been X-rayed – the bones were normal and the inference drawn was that nothing, therefore, could be wrong – quite false of course. It must be recognized that standard X-rays only give information as to whether disease is present or not in the vertebrae. Functional X-rays give more information about how the weight is distributed and whether tilting and faulty alignment is present, but even these do not give information about the soft tissues – the muscles, the ligaments, the nerves and the blood vessels.

Special tests   Should this information still fail to determine the cause of the symptoms it may be necessary to make special investigations. For example a myelogram may be needed to determine the size and shape of the spinal canal. Some back pains are due to, or at least accentuated by, the spinal canal being smaller than average (stenosed). The dye which is injected into the canal for a myelogram can show the dimensions and shape of the canal and a distortion of the shape will help in determining the cause of the pressure.

A tomograph is a special X-ray examination of the spine in which different sections of the vertebrae can be shown. This is very useful in diseased bone but diseased bone is a rarity and need only be considered by the orthopaedic specialist.

When spinal lesions, of whatever nature, cause abnormal changes in the nerves of the spinal cord or the nerve roots, special tests need to be carried out. Simple nerve tests are routine in a medical examination, but in complicated problems a neurologist may proceed with other special tests like a lumbar puncture to examine the cerebro-spinal fluid, or an electro-myelograph to record the conduction between nerves and the muscles. There are still other and newer scanning procedures which are mainly used for detecting tumours in the nervous system.

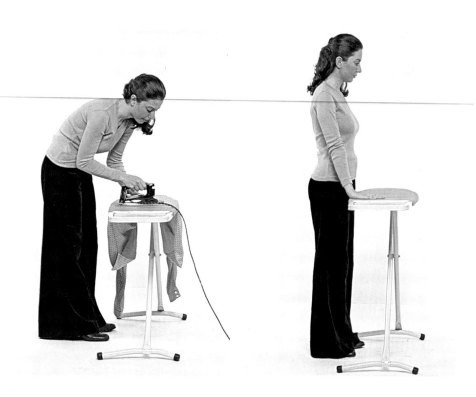

No need to bend while ironing. A straight back is far less tiring.

If your hand can be placed on a working surface without bending your arm or back, then it is the right height.

RIGHT: Making beds, can be a heavy job, particularly since you do it every day, and you may easily strain your back ... unless you kneel and take the weight on arms and shoulders instead.

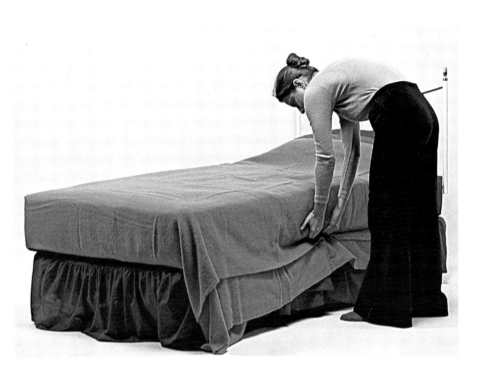

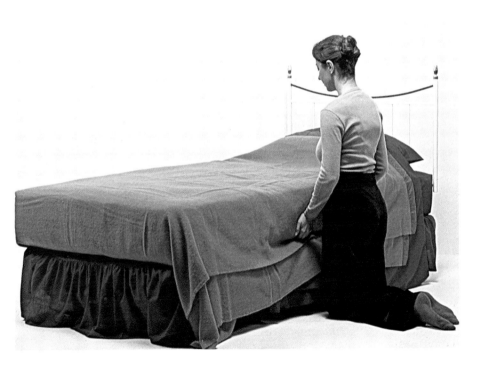

4 PREVENTION OF BACK PROBLEMS

Before dealing with treatment in a later chapter I want to make some suggestions for taking steps to reduce the risk of developing spinal pain long before the pain has started.

Heredity factors, congenital faults and growth disorders are outside anybody's control, but injuries, mechanical stresses and faulty posture can he modified or prevented to reduce the risk. In people with predispositions for back pain, some occupations should not be taken up.

Heredity plays its part and if your parents suffer from back problems then it is sensible, particularly if you are young, to make sure nothing is wrong.

Congenital faults are unavoidable in our present state of knowledge and some defects like spina bifida may be either so serious as to require surgery or so slight as to be ignored. Such defects may be obvious to a doctor or only discovered later when symptoms begin. One of the first symptoms of spina bifida is often a dimple in the middle of the spine in the lower lumbar region where it joins the sacrum. If you discover such a dimple consult a doctor. You will also need advice about taking up certain occuptions and adopting different sports.

Developmental faults are common in the spine (see page 47 where osteochondrosis is described). It is my view that all teenagers should be examined at least once between the ages of thirteen and twenty to see if they have any signs of osteochondrosis. If present then an assessment needs to be made, directing such young people into suitable occupations and outdoor activities as well as avoiding unsuitable ones.

Occupations which involve heavy lifting and bending, especially with a twisting component, should be avoided by all people who have congenital or developmental faults in their spines. At present these problems are being tackled and studies are being undertaken to identify those occupations which give greater risk to the spine. Only cursory medical attention is given at present to those people who are entering these occupations. Much more should be done to discourage those at risk from doing these jobs – and in the long run this would make economic sense because an injured worker becomes a liability to a firm rather than an asset.

Sport is a pastime for the majority and an occupation only for the few. Injuries to the spine are unavoidable when youth engages in competitive sports. We must not condemn the sport for this but greater care needs to be taken with medical examination and assessment following injuries so that further injuries are avoided. At least the risk should be explained and the possible outcome appreciated.

There is a practical difficulty here because some spinal injuries are not immediately apparent. For example a fall on to the base of the spine may do damage which does not cause pain at the time, nor cause any demonstrable X-ray changes. This is because discs have no nerve endings and interior disc damage can occur without pain. The only advice we can give to a person who has compressed his spine is that sufficient time for good repair should be allowed before taking risks again. The minor stiffness and aching following spinal injury ought to be taken more seriously than, say, the equivalent pain and stiffness in an injured limb joint.

The one sport I condemn wholeheartedly is professional *boxing*. In no other sport is it the express objective to injure the opponent. Even in karate and jiujitsu where damage can be inflicted the professed purpose is self-defence. Wrestling for entertainment 'value' is merely a show and does no harm to the participants. Proper wrestling is probably very beneficial as the competition itself is not intended to produce physical damage.

Soccer has its risks, but when played fairly there are no intentions to injure the opposition. The risks in soccer are much more to the legs than to the spine, whereas with rugby football and American football there are considerable compression forces on the spine. Rugby football should be avoided by anyone with congenital or developmental defects in the spine. The same goes for North American football. Any compression injury should be considered seriously not merely for the occasion but because of the later risk of disc degeneration and its attendant miseries.

With all other sports there are inevitable risks but we cannot stop them just for this.

Riding for example is a splendid exercise for the legs and spine. It is only the falling off which is risky! Similarly with skiing. Smooth even swinging at golf is free from risk but faulty technique or driving a ball hard out of a bunker can jar the spine unduly. There are twisting and bending components in squash, tennis, hockey, lacrosse, baseball, ice-hockey and cricket but it is only when movements are performed out of control that damage can occur.

Walking is a good symmetrical exercise, but for those with bad backs it is better to walk on grass than on hard paths or sidewalks because the springiness of the turf cushions the jarring effect of walking. Running and jogging should be done on the toes for the same reason. Heavy, repetitive landing on the heels jars the spine badly. Rubber soles and heels have a cushioning effect and there is less jarring of the discs.

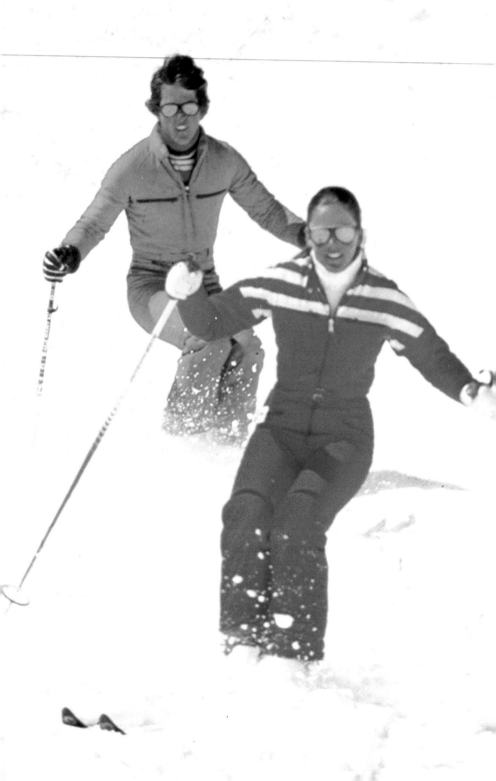

Sailing is an active sport but there are right and wrong ways of doing this too. Pulling down on halyards is beneficial because a stretching effect occurs in the spine, whereas heaving on the sheets with a bent back can compress the spine too much especially when the pulling is sustained. Capsizing is therefore not the only risk!

For the cruising man heaving in the anchor in unsettled weather can be risky but by having mechanical aids with winches and by housing the anchor outboard rather than inboard the effect and strain is reduced. Rowing should be done with as straight a spine as possible using the knees and hips to do the bending.

Fencing and bowling at cricket both jar the spine because of lunging, coming down heavily on one foot. Hang-gliding and parachuting have obvious risks but proponents teach the proper techniques of falling. In jiujitsu there is great emphasis on correct falling to minimize jarring.

Swimming is the sport I can recommend to all without reservation because the weight of the body and limbs is supported by the water. When swimming you can be as vigorous as you like without risk of straining joints in the spine. Occasionally a lordosis syndrome is accentuated by over-arching the spine with the breast stroke or by a bad dive when the legs flip backwards.

Young people can take greater risks than those over thirty-five years of age, but proper training in the chosen sport can lead to better performance and to a reduction in subsequent sprains. During training the muscles must be in control all the time and no attempt should be made to reach the impossible ball. Understandably in competitions the individual tries harder but over-reaching in uncontrolled fashion can do damage in even the best-trained athlete.

Balance is the key because, when in balance, the muscles on both sides of the centre of gravity can act to protect the spine. When off-balance it is better to let go than struggle to regain balance. Regaining balance can be at the expense of excessive muscle effort – tearing the muscles and ligaments. It is better to fall and sustain a bruise which takes less time to recover from than torn tissue. Alcohol reduces the risk of strain, but it does not improve performance so that is no answer!

In sexual intercourse only excessive or kinky methods cause any risk to the spine! Even where the spine of either party is faulty the risks of normal intercourse lying down are minimal. Pain in the spine may make sexual movements difficult and this must be recognized and is off-putting, but if any other position can be adopted without pain then sexual activity need not be avoided. After all the partner whose back is normal can do most of the moving when necessary. Intercourse involves flexing and extending the lumbar spine in the horizontal position with no vertical compression of the spine. Such movements are a good spinal exercise, and irrespective of whether sexual satisfaction is achieved or not we can at least say that the activity has been of benefit to the spine!

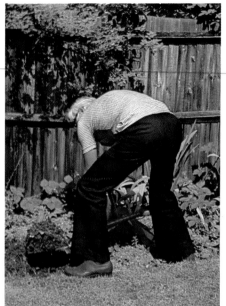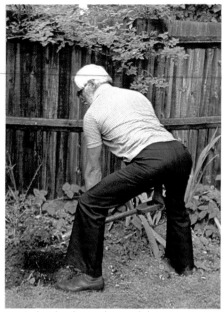

When digging don't stoop, its the quickest way to backache ... instead, keep your arms close to your body and let your trunk and legs take the weight.

Gardening is risky for those who have office jobs. Many such workers allow themselves to become flabby during the winter and they then go mad at gardening on the first warm weekend of spring. In some of the syndromes previously described it may be necessary to stop gardening altogether but in most cases it is possible to modify the method of gardening to reduce the risks. There are spades designed to help mechanical leverage and there are other mechanical aids, some of them motorized. The spit of soil on the spade can be halved. The wheelbarrow load can be reduced. The time spent at gardening can be cut down. Heavy work can be interspersed with lighter work. The length of the handle of the implement can be increased to reduce bending; getting close to the soil by going on to hands and knees will take most of the strain off the back.

After doing any sustained bending forwards the extension exercise (described on page 38) is worth doing. Hanging on a bar or bannister can help. Using the legs and knees to bend rather than bending the spine helps with wheelbarrow work – as does putting the load well forward in the wheelbarrow. In fact the weight should be well over the wheel itself to reduce the effect of the load to be lifted.

Keep whatever weight you lift close to your body rather than at a distance (above). It is worth making two journeys with half the load. It might take more time but it reduces the risk. Lifting more than 100 lb (45 kg) is unwise unless you are trained for the work. Do not forget the effects of lifting can be cumulative. You may lift 100 lb several times without risk, but if you keep lifting

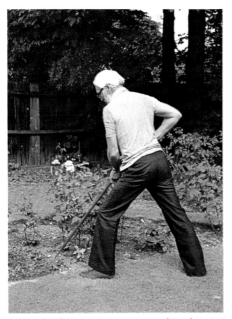
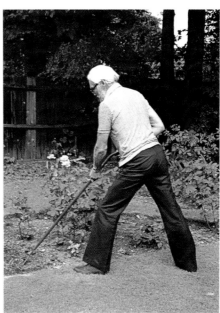

When hoeing use your arms rather than your back and keep balanced and upright.

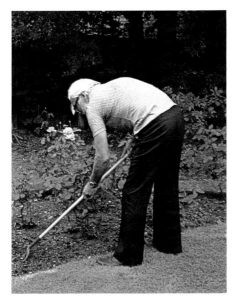
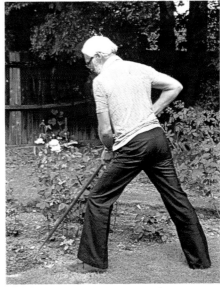

Bending over a hoe is a sure way to backache. The hoe should be long enough so you can stand upright, back straight, while working.

Standing upright is the way to hoe. Use your arms and shoulders, rather than your back, to do the work and keep balanced and upright at all times.

such a weight all day this can be disastrous. A bulky article (even of the same weight as a small article) will cause more strain because of the added stretch and leverage required. Lifting large boxes of groceries is a hazard in the same way as lifting a heavy load in the garden (pages 48–9 and 52–3).

When backache and stiffness develop it is more sensible to stop and do something else than to continue doing the same work. Building up muscle power (pages 85–91) will enable you to do more with less risk. When taking any strain, the muscles make the initial effort. If they are not strong enough, the ligaments are then strained and if the ligaments give way the load is increased on the discs. All movements should be performed under muscular control. Then, if the muscles are strong enough, the ligaments will not be damaged.

By and large direct injury to the spine is less damaging than indirect, because a direct blow to the spine merely causes bruising to the overlying tissues whereas indirect leverage can be severe enough to damage the ligaments and discs. A fall on to the tail may even fracture the coccyx but this effect is less significant than the transmitted jolt to the lumbar spine, just as a direct blow to the skull can fracture the cranium but the indirect jarring of the neck may have a more lasting effect.

5 EXERCISES AND POSTURE

In this chapter and the next I will outline the treatment which is available to you if you have a back problem. Since self-help is essential if your back is to recover fully – and to stay recovered – exercises and good posture are highly recommended and will be described here.

Exercises

Good muscle tone is the best safeguard against a repetition of back trouble. Exercises will help you if you have a mechanical spinal problem. Basically there are two types of exercise, one which stretches the joints for the purpose of increasing mobility and the other for strengthening the muscles. Both types of exercise are usually necessary and both give an indirect benefit to the body by increasing circulation in the muscles and the joints involved. The adoption of good postures whether sitting, standing or walking is an effort and in that sense correct posture is a form of exercise and will be described later.

Stretching exercises for the neck are best done separately rather than in combination.

1. It is better, and in elderly people it is safer, simply to stretch forwards, backwards, sideways, and to turn to each side separately (pages 70–73) rather than to combine them all together in one big circling movement. The stretch should be to the limit. If the limit of stretching is painful then advice should be obtained as to whether forcing the stretch into pain is desirable or otherwise. Some ten to twenty stretches in each of these six directions should be done.

2. There is an additional stretch exercise in the neck – the 'hen' exercise (page 73) – which is useful to move the upper thoracic joints. It is performed by moving the chin forwards and backwards in a horizontal plane rather like a hen does with each step it takes.
   The natural stiffening process of old age will accelerate if exercises are not done. If they are done regularly the rate of stiffening can be slowed down.

3. Stretching exercises for the thoracic and lumbar areas of the spine can be performed in six directions (pages 74–7), by reaching forwards towards the toes with the hands, arching backwards, reaching down sideways towards the knees with the hands to each side and turning left and right with the hands placed lightly on the hips. An exercise often done in the standing position,

The neck

Stretch your head forwards as far as it
will go and then stretch it backwards to
the limit. Avoid jerky, rapid movements.
Do this exercise slowly and rhythmically
without tension.

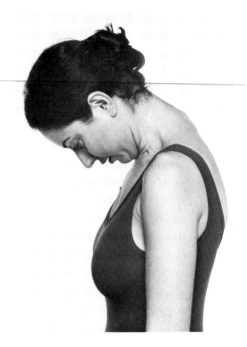

The neck

Side bend your head first to the left, then
to the right. Move it as far as it will go.

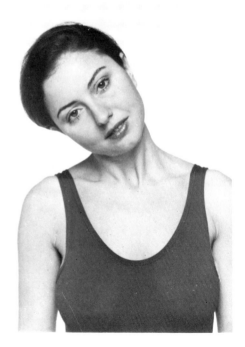

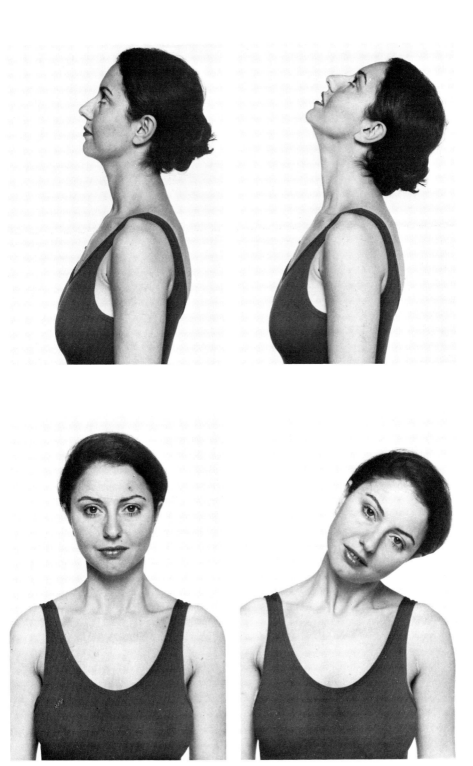

The neck
Turn your head to the left, then smoothly round to the right.

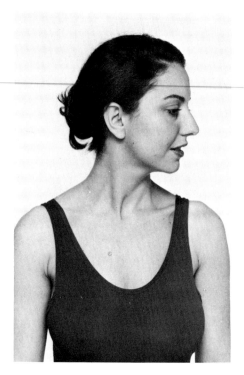

The 'hen'
Feel the joints in the spine move as you do this exercise. The joints which move are those between the neck and the thoracic spine.

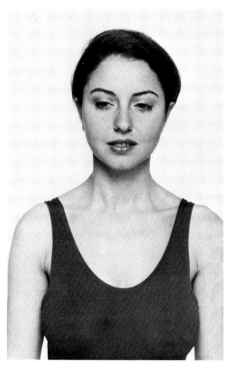
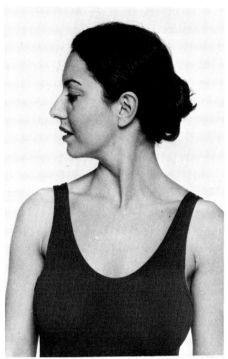
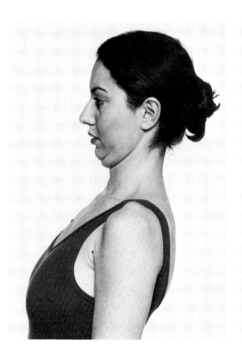
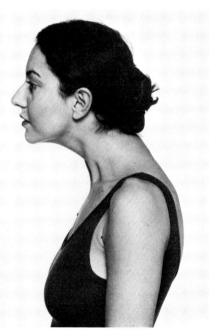

The back

The thoracic and lumbar areas of the spine can get quite stiff – unless you practise simple stretching. Lean backwards as far as you can go, then raise yourself to an upright position before touching your toes. If you cannot reach your toes stretch as far as is comfortable

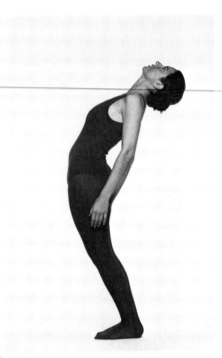

1

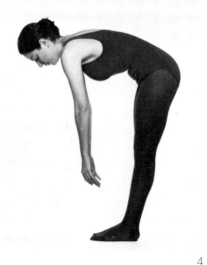

4

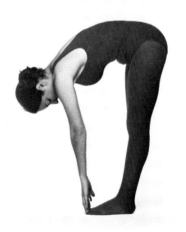

5

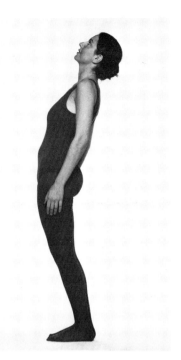 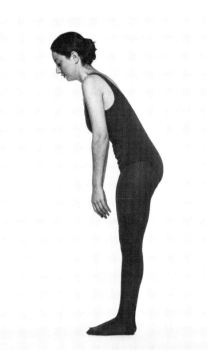

2   3

The back

When side bending take care not to push
yourself more than is practicable. Don't
bend forwards during this movement.

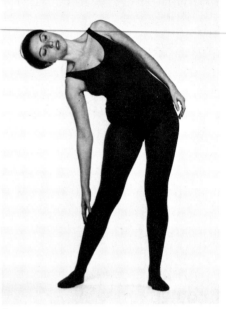

1

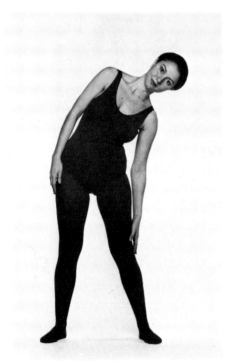

4

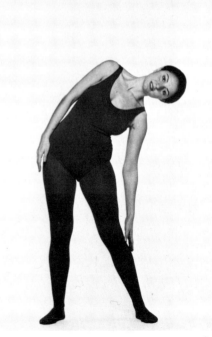

5

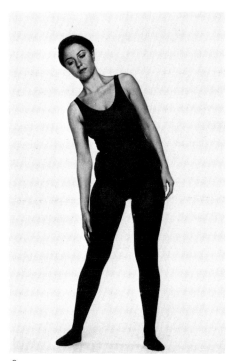

2

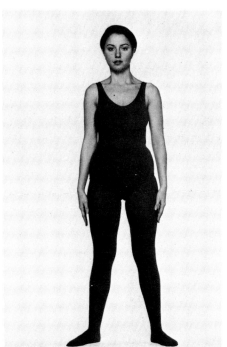

3

Breathing using arms

Stretch the thoracic spine by deep
breathing. Remember to breathe in
deeply as you raise your arms and
breathe out as the arms come forward.
Don't rush or you may get dizzy. Ten to
twelve very deep breaths are worth more
than hundreds of moderate breaths.

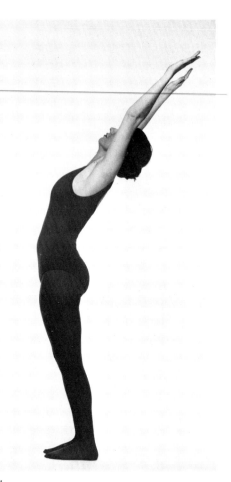

1

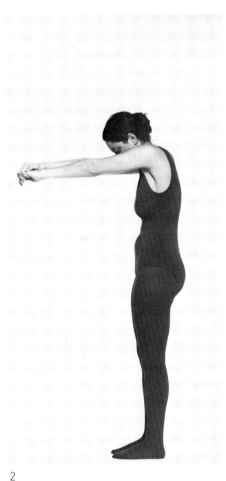

2

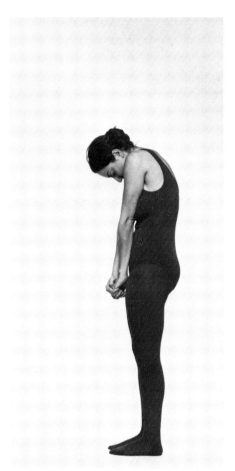

3

Breathing using hands

Begin this stretch for the thoracic spine by leaning forward. Start breathing in. Press your hands against your thighs to help breathing. Continue to breathe in . . . and in . . .

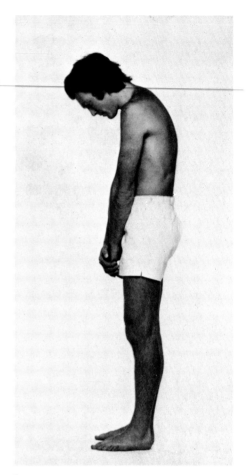

1

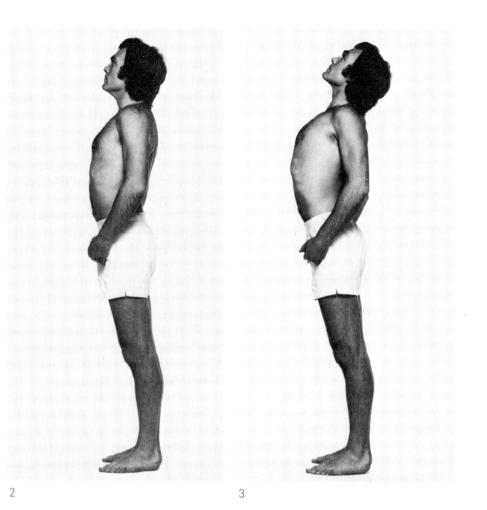

2   3

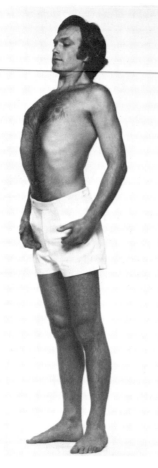

4

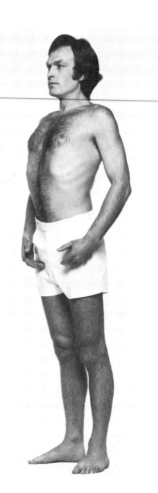

5

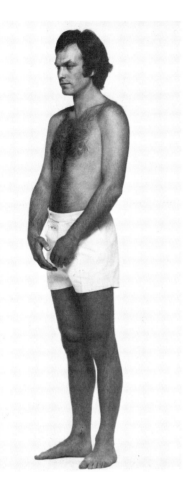

6

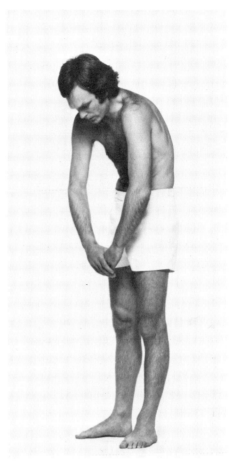

7 . . . until you can breathe in no more. Stretch your neck back at the same time. Let the air out gently and steadily and finish, head dropped forward. Repeat.

swinging the arms horizontally to left and right, can be overdone because the momentum of the arms may carry the body beyond its normal muscular control.

4. Another effective stretch for the thoracic spine is by deep breathing (pages 78–9). While standing, breath in deeply and reach up with the hands, arms fully stretched upwards and backwards, and arch the spine backwards. This is the best way of taking a deep breath. Then the arms should be brought down forwards, all the while breathing out as far as possible. The depth of breathing both in and out should be maximum and the arm movements help by forcing the ribs to expand fully and to contract fully. In doing so the thoracic vertebrae are also moved as well.

5. Another way to breathe deeply is to press your hands against your thighs while breathing in (pages 80–83).

6. The lower thoracic joints are effectively stretched by standing erect, holding the arms out sideways and at shoulder height, then reaching horizontally left and right. It is important to keep the pelvis stationary for this exercise. An observer watching the spine can see the effect on the spine at the junction of the thoracic and lumbar areas.

7. Lumbar movements can be increased in the same sort of way forwards, backwards, sideways and turning but in the presence of disc problems it is wise not to force the forward bending of the back. The other movements are safe. Bending forwards can be safely carried out when lying on the back and flexing the knees on to the chest (page 84).

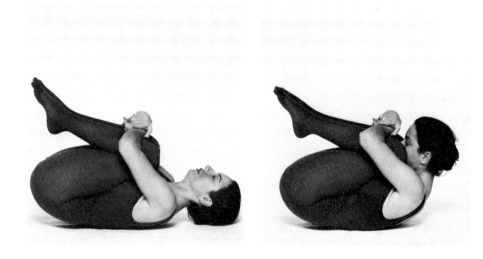

This is a safe way to bend. To increase the stretch bring your head up to your knees.

In yoga exercises where the emphasis is for maximum stretching, the spine can be disturbed by too much forward bending in the presence of disc lesions or where hypermobility and hypomobility occur in the same patient (page 25). The relaxation techniques and the majority of yoga exercises are safe and beneficial for most back problems.

Strengthening exercises   If you have a back problem, isometric muscular contractions are the safest and most effective way to build up muscle strength. By 'isometric' we mean that the muscle is contracted and is kept at the same length for a while. In other words, a position is adopted and that position is held by the muscular contraction. It is not the purpose of isometric exercises to contract the muscle to maximum power, rather it is to contract the muscle moderately. The sustaining of the effort and its repetition after pauses achieves the objective of increasing muscle power in a very effective and safe way.

1. The position for strengthening the whole of the posterior muscles of the spine is to lie face downwards (page 109), placing your hands down beside your body and lifting the head, shoulders and legs halfway up. The position should be held for ten seconds, then rest down for five seconds relaxing well in this interval, then rise again for ten seconds. Be content with six contractions the first day, eight the second day, ten the third and so on until you can do twenty of these ten-second lifts.

    The reason for not exerting maximum effort is that this would hyper-extend your spine, forcing the spinous processes together and causing discomfort if maintained. Your head and neck should be in line with the rest of the spine and not hyper-extended for the same reason.

2. The above exercise gives sufficient power for most purposes but, should you wish to increase power still further, place your hands on the top of your head and repeat the process (page 109). The latter exercise is much more strenuous and is as a rule not necessary.

    There are of course many modifications of this idea of isometric contractions and other ways are also effective for increasing muscle power but the simple exercises described here are easy enough to perform and not too time-consuming. Anybody with a back problem should be prepared to spend five minutes a day on keeping his muscles in good tone.

3. The most useful exercise for toning up abdominal muscles and to avoid risk to the spine is to lie on the back and move the legs as if riding a bicycle (pages 86–7). The lumbar spine should remain flat on the floor; elevate the legs well so that the thighs are at right angles with the floor. The cycling can be maintained for five minutes and if stronger abdominal muscles are required then the feet can be moved slowly further and further away as if the pedals of the bicycle were further from the tummy than before (pages 88–9). At maximum stretch this is a powerful exercise for the abdominal muscles. It should be avoided in people with lordosis problems (page 43). While the legs

Abdominal muscles
Start bicycling with short leg movements. Don't stretch too much.

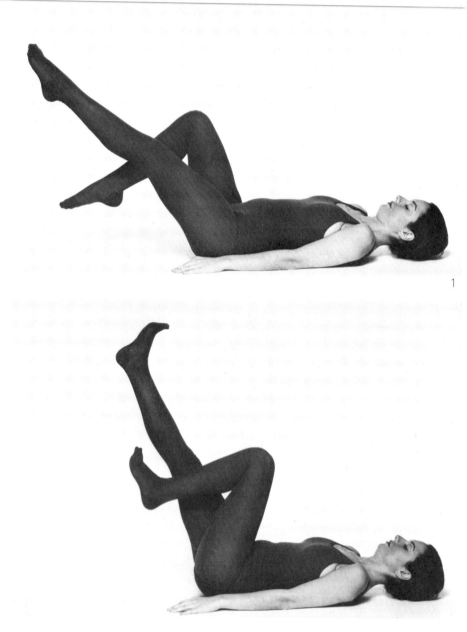

1

3

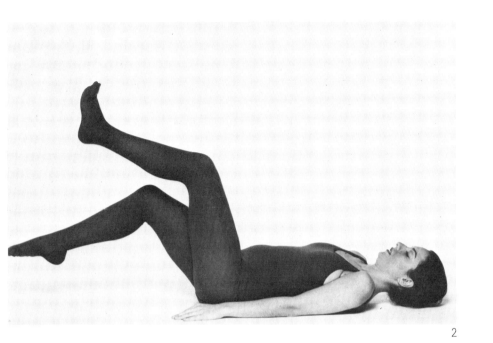

2

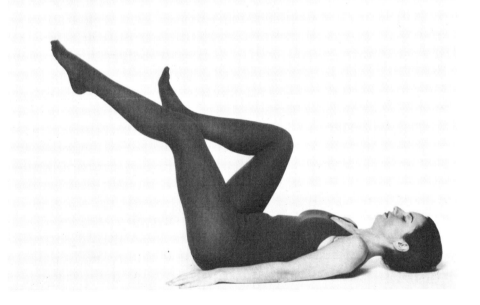

4

For stronger abdominal muscles push the toes away with a longer stretch.

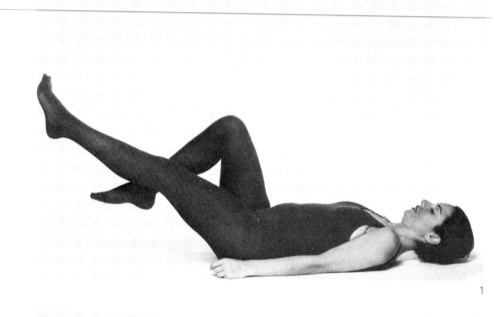

1

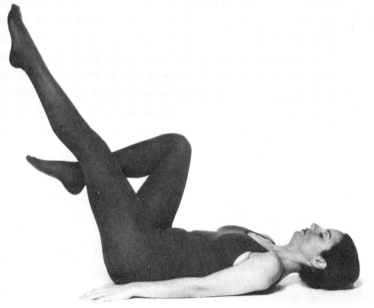

3

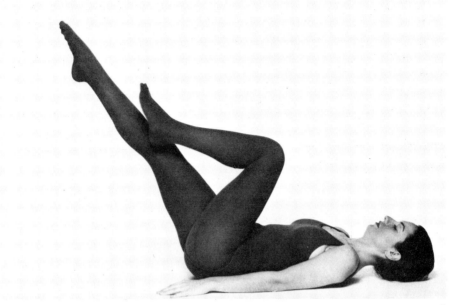

2

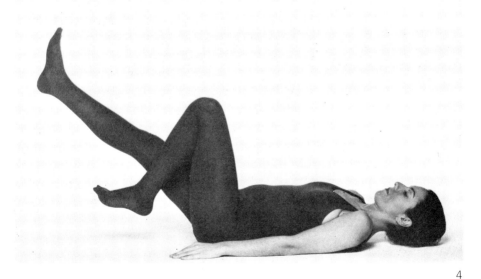

4

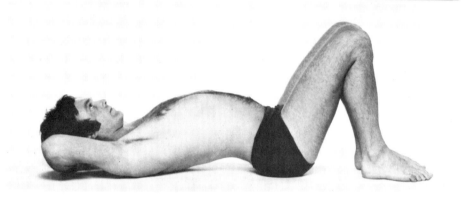

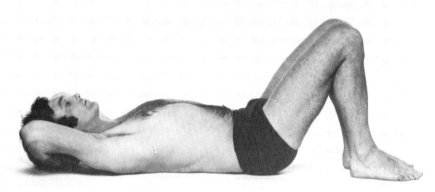

Another way to help a hollow back is to try flattening your spine so every part of your back touches the floor.

are performing the cycling movement the abdominal muscles are static, so that this exercise is still an isometric one for those muscles.

There are numerous other exercises which can be done with benefit but I have only described the basic and essential ones. I find that people are more likely to carry out instructions on exercises if they are simple and uncomplicated. There are, however, two other exercises which have particular application in people with hollow backs.

4. Standing with feet slightly apart to give stability, the pelvis is then tilted forwards (page 92). To do this it is not necessary to move the shoulders – if you find you are moving the shoulders then you are not performing the exercise correctly. The easiest way to think of this exercise is to think of the position of your bottom. In lordosis or hollow backs, the bottom 'sticks too far out' and to correct it the bottom must be 'tucked in'. Bottom out – bottom in – think of this and do not move the shoulders. You will then grasp what is required. The 'bottom in' position is a corrective position for lordosis and when standing this position should always be assumed. You will notice even if you do not think about it that when the bottom is 'tucked in' the abdominal muscles automatically contract. This is beneficial too to tone these muscles up during the exercise and during the adoption of this corrected position.

5. Another way to help correct a lordosis is to stand against a wall or lie flat (page 90). If you have a hollow back you will have difficulty in avoiding a space between the wall or the floor and the lumbar spine. The exercise then is to attempt to flatten the spine against the wall or against the floor.

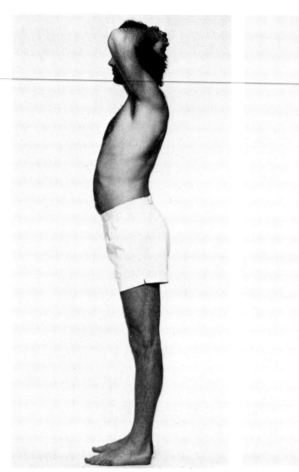
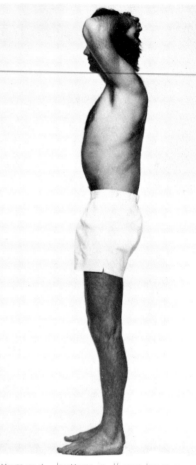

Bottom out – bottom in. If you have a hollow back (lordosis) this exercise will improve your posture. Remember to practise 'standing straight' during the rest of the day.

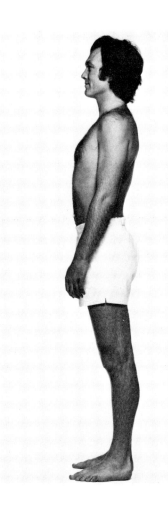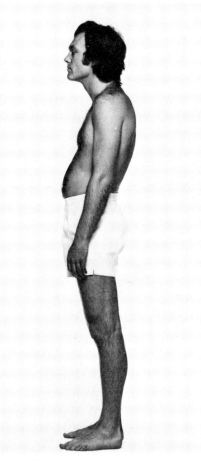

Stand tall, weight evenly distributed on both legs, head erect ... then deliberately slouch and sag. Notice what happens to your body (and mind!) when you do this.

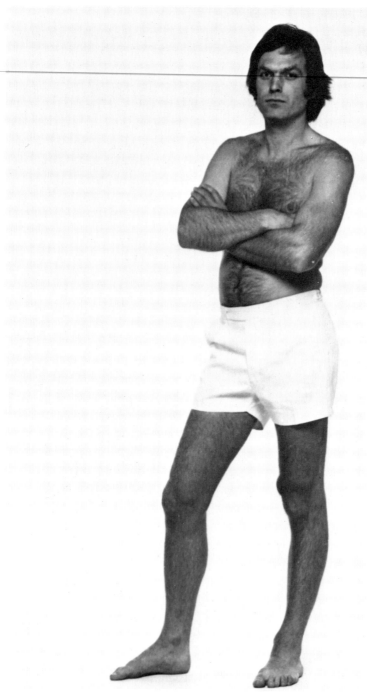

If you must take your weight on one leg (rather than on both) make sure it is not always the same leg.

Posture

Standing Good posture when standing is probably most easily achieved by the effort to 'stand tall' (page 93). This advice not only improves posture and good deportment but reduces the compression and sagging forces on the spine, the chest and the abdomen. Balancing a book or other object on your head is a good idea also, because it ensures that body weight is distributed evenly. Anyone can test this for themselves. Having tried to stand tall or balance a book on your head allow yourself deliberately to sag or slump into the sway posture (page 93). You will find that your shoulders droop, the abdomen bulges, the bottom sticks out and the curves of the spine all increase. The total height may diminish by 1 in (2.5 cm). There is of course extra effort required to regain that inch to stand tall, but not only does it look better but the abdominal organs are held up better. This improves the circulation there and reduces the risk of piles, constipation and prolapse. It is even more important for somebody who has a hollow back (lordosis) or round back (kyphosis) because the effort of standing tall diminishes the exaggerated curves of the spine.

Another sloppy posture which sometimes becomes a habit is taking the weight on one leg (page 94). This action reduces the total muscular effort of standing erect and puts a stretch on the ligaments of the leg which takes the weight and on the lower spinal ligaments. If the habit of standing on one leg is always to the same side those ligaments eventually protest and hurt but also there is a risk that a spinal curvature will develop. When prolonged standing is unavoidable it is safe enough to stand on one leg for a while, but swing over to the other side and give the first leg a rest too.

When attempting to stand tall the chin is kept in, the neck straightens, the shoulders ride naturally further back, the chest rises, the abdomen flattens, the lumbar spine straightens and the buttocks muscles contract. All these have good effects on the body generally and on the spine in particular.

Sitting posture is also important if only because many of us spend hours at a time sitting either at the office or at home. Sagging posture (page 100) can lead to the ligamentous strain syndrome (pages 28–30). Modern furniture design contributes to this problem as does the lack of parental and teacher guidance for the young. Sloppy posture when sitting is condoned. Parents and teachers set a poor example. It is partly a reaction to the rigid discipline of the Victorian era when children were expected to sit bolt upright and a stick was handy if the child got slack. Severe as it might have been, the system had its merit. No one heard about slipped discs at the beginning of the century! Back problems to a large extent stem from too much luxury – soft seats, soft beds and soft postures.

An exaggerated straight and upright position is not necessary but near vertical is best with the back rest of the seat supporting your spine to prevent sagging (page 100). The ideal *car seat* is one in which the back rest is adjustable not only in the upright position but also in the small of the back to give a greater or lesser bulge at the level of the lumbar spine. Volvo cars have adopted this system and their seats are very effective for virtually all back sufferers (page 57). The flat part of the seat should be long enough to give ample support to the thighs yet not too long otherwise the buttocks cannot reach the back rest.

The best way of sitting in a car seat is to lean forward, push your bottom as far back as possible and then place a cushion of suitable thickness into the lumbar spine before leaning back. There are back rests which can be placed in car seats to overcome the bad effects of 'luxury' seating and most of them have their protagonists, but the simple advice above is usually sufficient.

When covering long distances by car or truck you will notice, especially if you are the driver, that even though you make a conscious effort to sit well at the beginning of your journey you will tend to slump after a while even to the extent of finding it necessary to adjust the back view mirror. With good seating and adequate support this will not matter much but where the seat is too soft the driver will run a considerable risk of overstretching the lumbar ligaments. The effect of repeated journeys is cumulative unless the driver takes steps to counteract the bad effects of such posture (page 101).

Sleeping posture is not important except in soft luxury beds or when the spine is already a problem and painful. Much of the advertising done by firms selling beds is focussed on the mattress, but the mattress is far less important than the base. However well designed a mattress is, if it rests on a springy, sagging base the whole bed will then be a hazard to the sleeper. There is no need for any springs in the base whatsoever and a wooden structure is ideal. The mattress should be about 5 in (12 cm) thick and can be made from either foam rubber or springs. The foam rubber conforms to every shape and size; springs may also do so but not all mattresses are adequate in this way. The patient with a hollow or round back will require a more yielding mattress to accommodate the accentuated curves but the base should still be solid.

Where these types of beds are used it matters little whether you lie on your back, your front or on either side but when lying face down (prone) turn your head to one side. If such a position is held for too long, especially in the older person, pain and strain in the neck can follow. A modified prone position (page 97) will reduce some of the strain on the neck.

Prone lying can be an advantage in acute back pain because the circulation in the spine is better when prone – the blood drains away by the veins into the vena cava and back to the heart with the help of gravity. A change of position, however, is necessary several times during the night and most changes are done without even waking up. If the process of turning is painful then it is desirable to move the body as a whole from one position to another. You will need to make a conscious effort to do this but sleep need not be seriously disturbed. Turning on a sagging bed is more difficult and more painful than a firm one. If the bed sags a thick board should be placed between the mattress and the base. The wood should not bend even with two heavy people lying on it. A temporary measure is to place the mattress on the floor. If not possible then a pillow in the small of the back can minimize the sagging. If you have a hollow back you will find prone

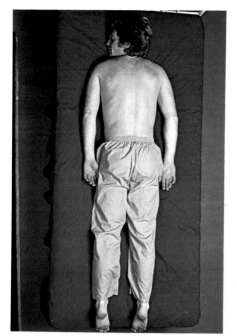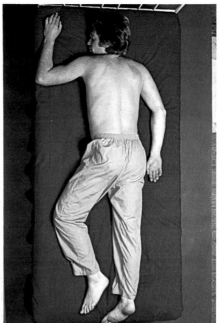

If you sleep on your front you may find it more comfortable to raise one arm and leg. There is less strain on the neck this way.

lying in a sagging bed the worst position you can adopt. You will find it better to be on one side with the knees and hips flexed up. In the same way if you suffer from sciatica you will often find a flexed position less painful and a cushion under the knee often gives relief.

Relaxation Many back sufferers would benefit from a rest in the afternoons – even ten minutes is worthwhile providing there is complete relaxation. The great advantage of lying down rather than sitting down to rest after lunch is that the discs are no longer compressed when the body is horizontal. Sitting relaxes the legs and spinal muscles, but still compresses the discs. Not everybody can relax well and practice of the art of relaxation is needed for most people. A useful method of relaxation is to lie on the back on the floor with a low pillow and commence the process of 'letting go' at the feet first, gradually working upwards to the head. The idea is to think of the muscles area by area – feet, calves, thighs, bottom, abdomen, chest, hands, arms, shoulders, neck and face in that order. Ask yourself, thinking of each area in turn, whether the muscles are completely floppy or not. If not you tense the muscles and then let go. Finally think of your eyes to make sure the lids are relaxed. Then let the mind go blank and relaxation is then complete. Many will find it difficult to achieve full relaxation but with practice most people can manage it. The time taken to achieve full relaxation can be shortened with practice until it is almost instantaneous. Even sleep can be achieved rapidly with this technique after much practice. There is a companion book to this one, *Stress and Relaxation* by Jane Madders, and if you have difficulty in relaxation you would benefit from her advice.

The majority of simple back problems can be resolved if proper attention is given to the postures of standing, sitting and lying, together with adequate exercise to maintain good muscle tone in the spinal muscles, and allocating sufficient time for rest and relaxation.

6 HOW DOCTORS AND THERAPISTS CAN HELP YOU

Methods of treatment

Prevention is better than cure but if you have already got a spinal problem some of the treatments currently available to you are as follows:

1. Manipulation
2. Massage
3. Traction
4. Collars and corsets
5. Sclerosing injections
6. Electrotherapy
7. Hydrotherapy
8. Drugs
9. Surgery and other methods

Exercises, which are both preventive and curative, have been described in the last chapter.

Manipulation

I place manipulation at the head of the list of treatments of the spine because it has almost universal application. In some conditions manipulation is harmful but when properly applied and in the appropriate case, manipulation is the most effective single method of available treatments. The term manipulation needs explanation, however, because there are various schools of thought with differing ideas and you will need to be cautious about going to the right practitioner for manipulative treatment.

The schools of manipulation are: osteopathic, chiropractic, orthopaedic and bone setting.

Bone setting goes back in history further than the other methods and there were famous bone setters like Sir Herbert Barker in London, England. Bone setters developed their skills through apprenticeship and intuitive ability. The techniques were applied rather by the rule-of-thumb method than from diagnosis – all the patients tending to receive the same technique without scrupulous analysis of the mechanical problem.

Orthopaedic surgeons watching bone setters observed the benefits of the treatment and adopted the techniques, applying them with more medical

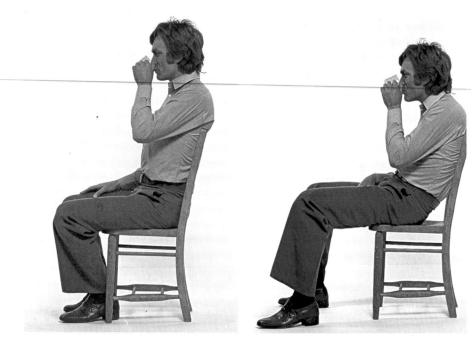

When sitting keep upright. A slumped position eventually leads to backache.

If you are working at a desk make sure you have proper back support and raise the working surface to avoid sagging.

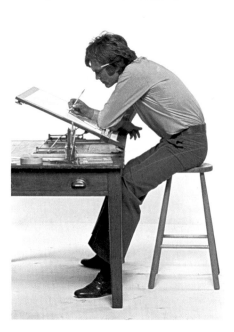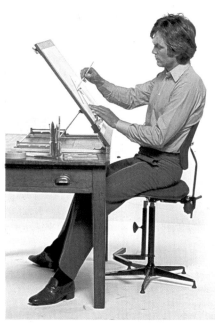

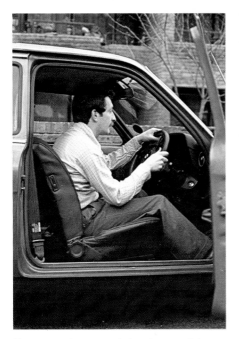

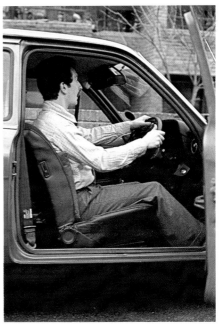

No way to have a painless journey! A slouched, hunched posture will always end in an aching back.

The same car but this time lumbar support helps maintain a good, balanced posture.

knowledge and withholding manipulation in the presence of disease. The tendency grew for the orthopaedic surgeon to manipulate only for adhesions and only with the help of an anaesthetic and only forcing the affected joints through their maximum range to ensure full mobility in the restricted joints. This is a limited application for manipulation. Furthermore most manipulations do not require an anaesthetic. There are, however, some conditions which do require anaesthesia. The osteopathic profession has developed techniques and skills which are a considerable refinement on the orthopaedic approach.

Osteopathy was started over one hundred years ago by A.T. Still in Missouri, USA. He worked out techniques based upon a study of anatomy and leverages. His followers grew more skilled with continuous application. After all, if manipulation is the only method used then the practitioner acquires greater skills than the part-time practitioner who is spending most of his time in other skills. Surgery is one of the greatest of all manual skills and takes many years of study and application to perfect. It is better therefore for the orthopaedic surgeon to devote his hard-earned skills in that area rather than in manipulation. The osteopath in the UK and Canada devotes all his time to patients who benefit from manipulation and he rejects those patients for whom manipulation is not appropriate and therefore he will develop his techniques to greater effect. Osteopathic techniques are modified according to the mechanical diagnosis and if disease is present then manipulation is not performed on such patients.

As previously stated there are many causes of back pain and manipulations of mechanical faults are varied and numerous. It is the duty of the osteopath to analyse each case as precisely as he can because such precision is necessary for the application of the correct and appropriate techniques.

Obviously a wide medical background of anatomy, physiology and pathology are prerequisites for osteopathy and it would be ideal if all had medical degrees, but with the full training provided, say, by the British School of Osteopathy patients are safeguarded against injudicious, inappropriate and excessive manipulation. In the USA a licensed osteopath has had full medical training and in Canada a license is awarded to those who have qualified in the US or UK. A skilled osteopath can, by correct use of leverages, manipulate any single joint in the spinal column and in this way can apply the manipulation accurately to the affected joint. Such refinements of techniques are not taught in medical schools and until the day comes when such skills are imparted to medical students there will always be a place and a demand for osteopathy.

The chiropractic school was an off-shoot from the osteopathic, and chiropractors tend to use more direct force on the vertebrae themselves rather than on using the leverage techniques of the osteopath. Chiropractic techniques when not abused have great merit. Skilled manipulators tend to use methods from all the schools where appropriate.

Manipulation in the broadest sense is not just a single manoeuvre applied at one

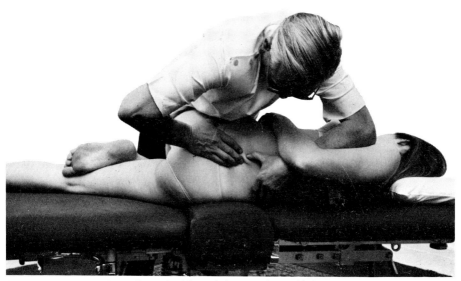

Twisting manipulation relieves locking of the apophyseal joints.

site on one occasion, because it can be given repetitively and gently thereby having a persuasive effect rather than a harsh forced effect. Much of the osteopath's time is spent in rhythmic, repetitive movements to encourage better mobility in the affected joints rather than by using extreme force on one occasion.

By and large an osteopathic treatment consists first of the mechanical assessment, followed by treating the muscles and ligaments, using massage, stretching, articulation and traction, and then, finally, if the joint will not yet move freely, by a specific thrusting technique to release the joint fixation. The osteopath is not 'putting a bone into place' after it has been displaced, rather is he freeing or releasing the relative fixation in the joint. He releases the 'bind' or the adhesions which are preventing full mobility. The manipulations may need repeating on several occasions, not because in the interval the bone has gone out again but because the joint has stiffened once more.

These techniques are particularly appropriate in the commonest of syndromes described earlier, namely, the adhesions syndromes. They are not applicable to the ligamentous strain syndromes and the techniques have to be modified considerably in the episodic, degenerative and inflammatory syndromes as was previously stated.

Probably the best way to choose a manipulator is by reputation. The skilled operator will have a good reputation, the unskilled an indifferent one. Proper qualifications anywhere in the world are the best safeguard. For example, a registered osteopath in the UK has to have had a full-time four years' training and has to abide by high professional codes of conduct equivalent to those of the medical profession. Practitioners who infringe these codes are suspect and the public should be wary of them.

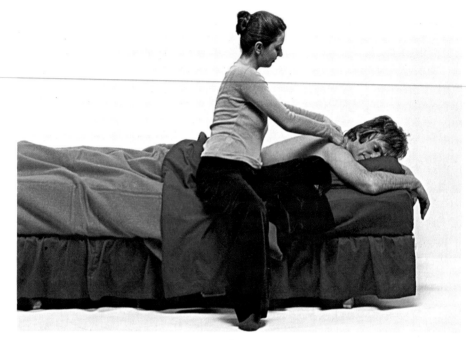

Massaging aching muscles can be helpful and enjoyable. Be careful not to dig in the tips of your fingers and thumbs. Short fingernails are essential!

The illustrations (pages 103 and 106) are examples of typical specific manipulations frequently used in osteopathic treatment.

Massage

Massage is a method of treating muscles and other soft tissues in the body and it has important applications especially in the soft tissue syndromes described earlier. The Swedish massage school was in great vogue between the First and Second World Wars but tended to lose popularity during the Second World War because young recruits and injured young people did not need it.

Not everybody can benefit from general exercise programmes. Then individual detailed attention is necessary. Furthermore, if you are elderly you may be quite unable to undertake strenuous physical exercise and massage and manipulation becomes necessary.

Massage is frequently an essential preliminary treatment before manipulation is done, because tense and contracted muscles can interfere with effective manipulation. In addition the massage will help you to relax better.

As a rule massage is applied together with, or following, the application of heat. This is because heat itself helps to relax the muscles and facilitates the massage. Nevertheless, merely to massage tight muscles without dealing with the cause of the tightening will of course give only temporary benefit. Pleasant

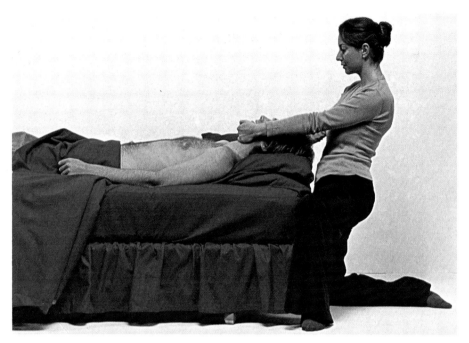

It is quite safe to give traction so long as you receive instructions from your doctor on how to do this. But do get advice – otherwise you could inflict damage.

though massage is (and effective at the time) it will have but a transient effect if causes are not eradicated. Massage cannot disperse fat except on the operator! The hard panniculitis described earlier (page 50) can be softened with vigorous massage but, if you have such a condition, you must reduce weight to achieve a lasting response.

Liniments can be used. Their purpose is that of mild skin irritation. It has been found that irritating the skin can alter the pain sensations in deeper structures. This applies of course only if the pain is moderate. To be effective the liniment must redden your skin. The irritant provokes a histamine response and the superficial blood vessels dilate thereby increasing the circulation to the skin and even improving the blood supply to deeper structures.

Traction

This method of treating spinal problems has had its advocates and has been in vogue in the last few years, but its universal application has now ceased.

There are several ways in which the spine can be stretched and each of them has its merits and disadvantages. To condemn the method entirely is just as bad as applying it to all-and-sundry back problems. The diagnosis has to be made and the right form of traction applied.

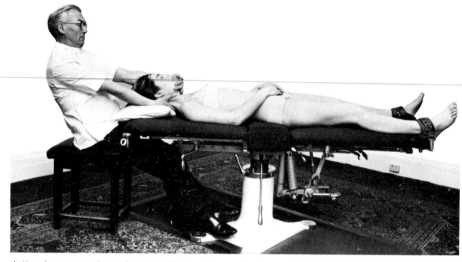
Adjustive manual traction can help a disc protrusion.

Sustained traction means that the patient is strapped in two places in the spine depending upon which area is affected. For the neck it is usual to apply a halter round the chin and back of the head. The halter is attached to cords and a spreader, and then through a balance (for measuring the amount of traction) to weights or to apparatus. The traction force may vary from 10–70 lb (4.5–32 kg) depending upon the size of patient and the amount required to give relief. The traction can be sustained but should only be given where nerves are being compressed and if the traction is effective in relieving the pain. Naturally the traction has to be done under medical supervision. The pull may be horizontal or vertical but a vertical pull largely defeats the objective because it forces the neck backwards and this prevents opening of the foramina in the neck and so fails to achieve effective separation. Horizontal traction, using a pillow to flex the neck slightly, is better and is in any case pleasanter and more acceptable for the patient.

Intermittent sustained traction is applied as before but the pull is only maintained for half a minute at a time and repeated several times. The optimum pull for such traction is 35 lb (16 kg). The advantage of intermittent traction is that the ligaments are not over-stretched and the circulation is encouraged rather than stagnating as must happen when sustained traction is applied.

Rhythmic traction is ideally used for degenerating discs which are not causing nerve-root-pressure symptoms. The purpose is to encourage the flow of tissue fluid between bone and cartilage by a gentle rhythmic pulse of stretch and relaxation. The results of rhythmic traction are only slowly apparent because the effect is indirect on the circulation to the spine. It is, however, the only effective way I know of influencing the circulation to the discs (page 21).

106

Adjustive traction is a technique of manipulation which should only be used by a skilled operator. It is applicable when a disc is bulging though not displaced. A reduction in the bulge is possible and the method is very effective when everything tallies – the right time, the right patient, the right condition and the right operator. If this technique is unsuccessful it is free from risk in skilled hands so it has a very important place in the range of treatments.

Collars and corsets

In acute syndromes where pain is accentuated by movement external support can give great relief by reducing such movements either in the neck or the back using a collar or a corset. In severe cases it is necessary to immobilize the spine completely in a plaster-of-paris jacket or collar, but in most cases a plastic collar (page 29) which is very lightweight and does not stop all movements is sufficient. Similarly, a corset (page 29), having reinforcing bars which fit well into the lumbar curve and with velcro fittings in front, is adequate to provide some support and to check excess movement. Collars and corsets used when the acute symptoms are present will help the pain to subside.

Making your own   A home-made collar (see below) can be made by rolling several sheets of newspaper from corner to corner in such a way that the middle is thicker than the ends. The roll of paper is then flattened so that it is about 5 in (12 cm) wide. This is applied to the back of the neck and the tapering ends are

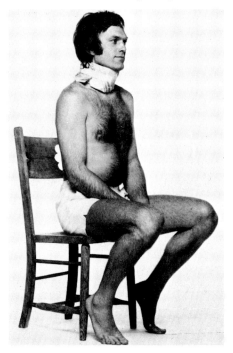

A home-made collar, easy to construct, gives support to the neck.

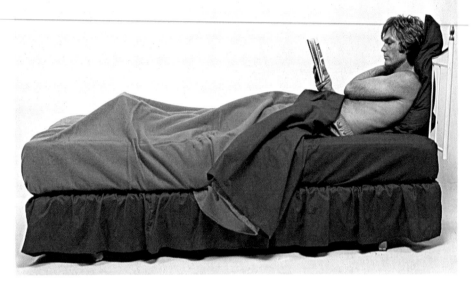

Reading in bed may seem like a good idea but, however many pillows you have, your back will not enjoy it.

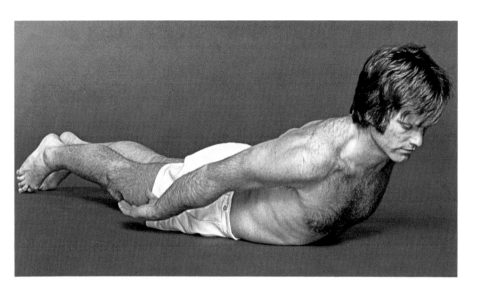

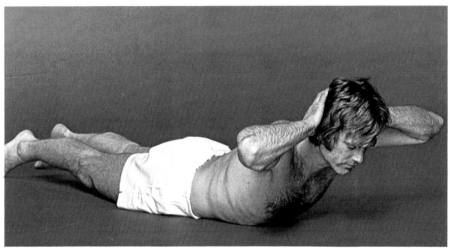

This is a strenuous exercise for strengthening the back muscles (see page 85). Don't raise your head and neck too far; excessive arching sometimes causes pain.

folded round at the front of the neck. The whole paper collar can be softened with a cravat or scarf. This device will not support your neck much but it is better than nothing. It can be easily renewed and reinforced as necessary. The support should be so arranged as to check backward bending. In most acute neck complaints the attempt to bend backward accentuates the pain and it is better to hold the neck slightly forwards from the erect position. A similar and better home-made collar can be achieved using 1 in (2.5 cm) sorbo rubber and stockinette.

It is not so easy to devise a home-made corset but it is surprisingly helpful to apply 2 in (5 cm) adhesive strapping (non-stretch variety) to circle the back and abdomen. Two long strips at the back reaching from the shoulders to the buttocks also restricts because the stripping adheres to the hairs of the skin and bending forward pulls and reminds the person not to bend further!

The use of collars and corsets should be limited to a maximum of six weeks. If they are used longer than this the muscles of the spine will begin to rely on the support and they become weaker unless you do active isometric exercises (pages 85–91).

Sclerosing injections

This is a method of injecting ligaments and is designed to reinforce weak ligaments (pages 28–30). (Sclerosing literally means hardening but firming is what is achieved in this context.) The chemical used is ethanolamine oleate which has long been used for the injection of varicose veins to tighten them up. It acts by irritating the tissues, setting up an inflammatory response which in turn leads to fibrous tissue formation. As ligaments are made of fibrous tissue the new fibres reinforce the old and a lasting repair can be achieved. These fibres are natural to the body – not some extraneous artificial aid – and are therefore more acceptable. Another formula for sclerosing injections is a combination of phenol and glucose. This sclerosing method was started in the fifties by Hackett in America and, although not a universally adopted method, the response to these injections is excellent. If you have strained ligaments you may benefit from sclerosing injections; this treatment is also useful in disc degeneration because instability is part of the process of degeneration.

Electrotherapy

There are several electrical treatments, namely, short-wave, diathermy, micro-wave and ultrasonic therapy. Their purpose is to increase circulation. They have limited application to the spine, but if you have arthritis these treatments are helpful even though not curative.

Electrical methods of heat production have their use too, because any form of heat helps to relax tense and painful muscles. The advantage of electrical infra-red is that it can be maintained at a constant temperature. Electric infra-red lamps have no special merit compared with, say, hot-water bottles except that the rays can be localized better and the heat remains constant. The most convenient form of heat is a miniature electric blanket and this can be applied directly to the skin or even over clothing. The temperature can be adjusted to give maximum heat short of burning and the blanket can wrap round the afflicted area conveniently (page 37). The heat should be applied for fifteen to twenty minutes and can be repeated several times a day. Even though the benefit of heat is temporary it is worth having during recovery and while other methods are being used to resolve the underlying problem.

There is a recently introduced electrical stimulation which may well be helpful for back pain which has not yielded to other methods. The apparatus is called a transcutaneous nerve stimulator (TNS). The underlying idea is that an alternative stimulus to that of pain will often mask the pain and reduce it. The principle of counter-irritation has been used from time immemorial. (Similarly, with acupuncture, the needles create an alternative stimulus which in some way reduces the pain level.) The TNS apparatus stimulates on the skin instead of puncturing it. The efficacy of the apparatus has yet to be evaluated.

Hydrotherapy

Hydrotherapy is similar to electrotherapy in that it provides heat and comfort but is of no great lasting value. I have already mentioned the virtues of swimming. Sometimes jets of water are played on the spine but this is more a mechanical effect than a water effect.

Drugs

Drugs are well down on the list of treatment for back pain because I prefer to advocate natural methods of healing and because the major causes for back pain are mechanical and drugs merely have a chemical effect. In the severest of pains it may be justifiable to use morphine. In less severe cases drugs like pethidine, DF 118, aspirin, paracetemol, tylenol, robaxisa, etc., have a place if you must continue your work despite pain – but they have no curative value. In some inflammatory states the anti-inflammatory drugs like butazolidine and indocid are useful to tide a patient over a temporary inflammatory state, but they can have nasty side-effects such as indigestion and anaemia. Injections of local anaesthetics are helpful sometimes. A general anaesthetic to facilitate manipulation is occasionally necessary.

In these limited ways drugs may be useful but the underlying mechanical disorder needs mechanical methods to put it right, not chemical ones.

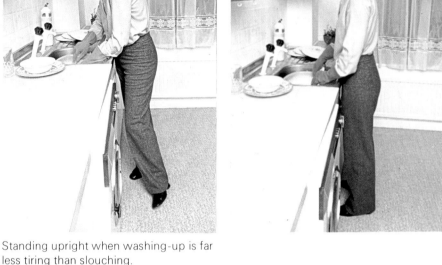

Standing upright when washing-up is far less tiring than slouching.

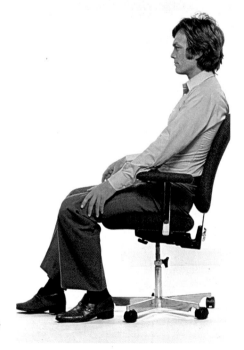

If you have a job which entails a lot of sitting, choose your chair carefully to give maximum lumbar support.

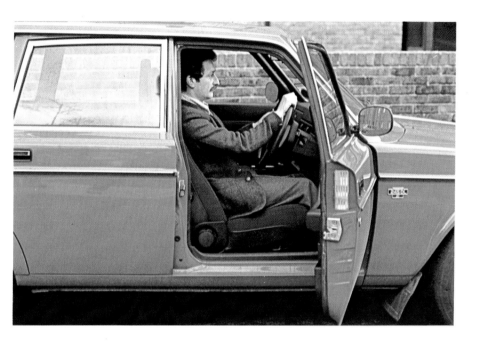

For the sake of your back if you have to drive often and for much of each day, choose a car with a well-designed seat as shown *above*. If you have no alternative an inexpensive way of providing lumbar support is to place a cushion in the small of your back.

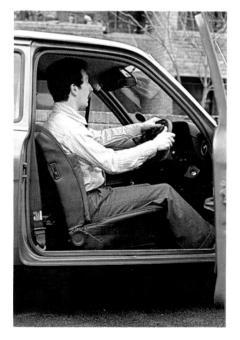

Surgery and other methods

We finally come to surgery, needed in a minute number of back problems: the intractible and large disc protrusion, the extremely unstable spine, the severe spondylolithesis, the serious spina bifida, the cases where pressure within the spinal cord is such that it interferes with the nerves and/or spinal cord, the rare cases of spinal cord tumours and bone tumours.

If you have to undergo surgery it will probably be one of two types. A laminectomy is the commonest of the surgical operations and this consists of removing a piece of lamina (fig. 4). This is done merely to facilitate the operation and give better access to the spinal canal where a disc displacement is causing obstruction to the nerve roots. The obstructing piece is removed and the soft centre of the disc is scooped out to stop any more displaced fragments from that disc. The divided muscles and skin are stitched together again.

In some instances a bone-grafting operation is justified so that further problems can be avoided in future. The objective is to fuse two or more vertebrae together and form a bony union. If successful the bony union stops all further movements at that level and thereby stops all displacements there in the future. The long-term worry about those patients (even with successful bony fusion) is that more stress is placed on the joints and vertebrae above. Those joints are thereby made more vulnerable to further mechanical stress.

Are there any other methods available to help back sufferers? There are, of course, advocates for acupuncture, hypnosis, psychotherapy, homeopathy, diet. These methods have been used with benefit, but as the majority of back problems are mechanical in origin they should be treated by mechanical means.

Diet can play its part in two ways. If you are overweight (causing mechanical effects) then calorie restrictions to a very low level can reduce your weight effectively – but this is not the place for a full discussion of weight reduction. The other factor in diet is the quality of the food – the need to have an adequate intake of fresh foods rich in vitamins and minerals, the need to have adequate roughage and the need to cut down on animal fats and proteins. The chemistry of cartilage is still not known except that it contains proteins and carbohydrates. Vitamin C is vital to the healthy metabolism of all connective tissues including cartilage. Bone metabolism is better understood nowadays and one cause of spinal pain later in life is osteoporosis when the bones become more porous and less calcified. Such people need extra calcium and vitamin D, not forgetting the other chemistry of bone – magnesium, phosphates, carbonates. It has been shown that vegetarians living on a high salad and vegetable intake are much less prone to osteoporosis than meat eaters, so a vegetarian diet is something to consider.

Anxiety is a factor in all medical problems – naturally enough because ill-health is a threat to happiness, comfort and secure living. Anxiety caused by back pain is particularly significant because the spine is so vital to mobility. If the cause of the back pain can be resolved and the pain relieved, anxiety in a normal person is also relieved. There are, however, many cases where mechanical faults are minimal and the anxiety state or the depressed state is dominant. Then the psychological factors which are creating the disturbed psyche must be dealt with otherwise the spinal condition will persist and a vicious cycle established. Ideally, treatment for the mechanical problem should be pursued at the same time as the causes for anxiety or depression are being treated.

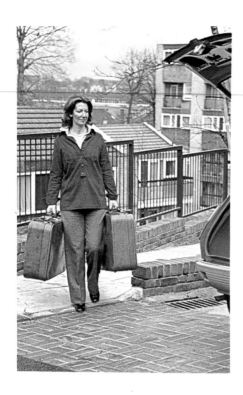

If you have a load to carry always try to balance your body. With suitcases, always carry two small ones rather than one large, heavy suitcase.

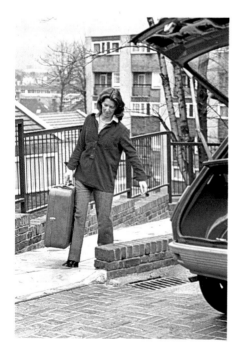

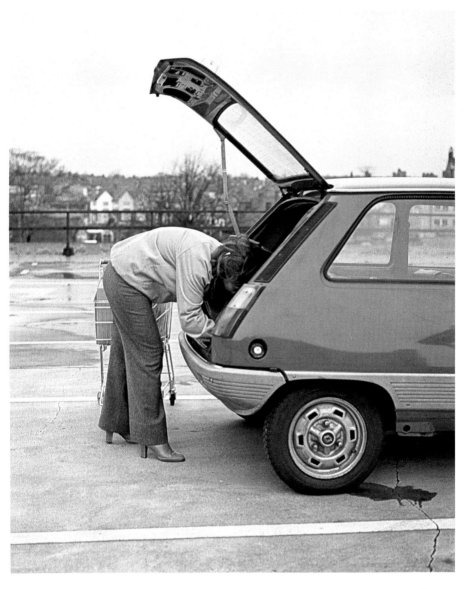

You could do yourself an injury by bending over with a heavy box of groceries. If you keep your back straight you won't come to much harm.

7 PRACTICAL HINTS TO PREVENT BACK PAIN

Below are listed some useful points to remember in reducing the risk of back strain. This summary complements the preventive measures discussed throughout the book.

Stand tall (page 93).

Do not weight bear on one leg for too long at a time (page 94).

Avoid any sustained bending forwards (page 100).

Arrange any bench work (and this includes kitchen surfaces, ironing, washing, etc.) at the correct height. This height for you can easily be found by standing against the bench, and relaxing the arm. The correct height of the bench for you is at wrist level (page 60). It is better on the whole for the bench to be too high than too low.

Sit with adequate back support (page 100).

When lifting any weight keep the weight close to your body. Keep the back as straight as possible. Use your hips and knees to bend rather than your back (pages 42–43).

Avoid, like the plague, a combination of lifting and twisting with a bent back (page 119). This is probably the most severe mechanical stress you can put on your back.

If you have to sneeze, sneeze upwards rather than downwards! Arch your back backwards when coughing.

Carry two small suitcases rather than one heavy one (pages 42–43).

If you have to lift repeatedly keep each lift to a reasonable minimum even if this takes twice as long.

Use mechanical devices where possible for lifting.

Supermarket shopping is a hazard in modern life because of the tendency to overload the basket. It is sensible to transfer the food into a basket on wheels and, when lifting the goods into the car (pages 52–53), great care should be taken especially if the angle is awkward. It is far better to take time unloading individual articles than to lift a whole box of groceries at once. Five minutes of this may save five days in bed.

Don't sag or slump (page 100).

Choose a chair which is the right height for you so that you can avoid leaning forwards all the time (page 100).

Choose a car by its seat and not by the engine (page 57).

Compensate for badly designed seats with firm pillows in the small of the back to prevent sagging (page 101).

Avoid chairs whose horizontal surface is too long for your thighs.

Refrain from sitting in deck chairs.

Don't get your back cold; this means that, if you find yourself sweating, cool down slowly rather than rapidly.

Golfers should use a trolley and limit the load to six clubs if a trolley is not available. Walk round the course unless your heart is weak.

For neck sufferers avoid heavy lifting, pulling and pushing strains. Keep away from painting the ceiling (page 56) and star gazing. Don't reach too high (page 120). Use firm pillows and avoid prone lying.

Counteract nervous stresses by relaxation and outdoor exercise. Swim every week.

Look after your back and your back will look after you – that's the message of this book. Your back is strong and perfectly capable of holding you up, without complaining, for the whole of your life. Treat it well and you need never suffer from back pain again.

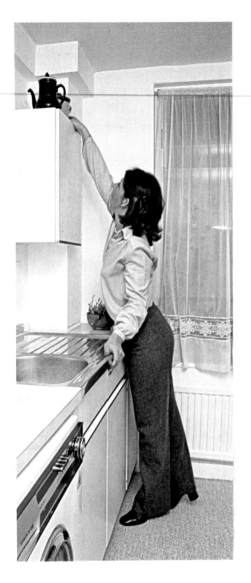
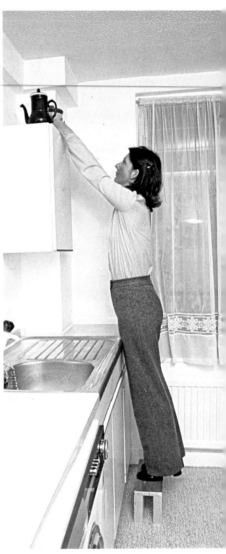

It is much safer and less of a strain to step up on to a stool to reach something from a high shelf. You can also see what you're doing!

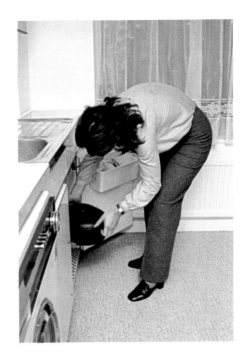

Twisting your back when you bend only adds insult to injury as your back is most vulnerable if you twist and bend at the same time as you lift. When getting a heavy casserole out of the oven bend at the knees and keep your back straight.

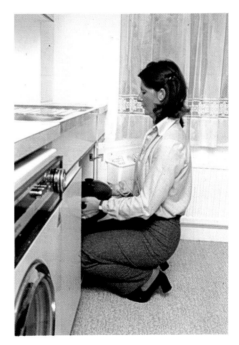

Acknowledgements

I would like to thank my son Malcolm who modelled so patiently for some of the exercises and postures. I also want to thank the other models, Agape Stassinopoulos and Evelyne Duval, together with the photographers, Simon Farrell and Bill Ling.

Thanks also to Rosemary Pettit who helped edit the manuscript, Mel Saunders who designed the book and Martin Dunitz who inspired the project.

Alan Stoddard

The publishers would like to thank: Mines and West for the Utopia Universal Chair (p. 112) and the Omnia Draftsman's Chair (pp. 6, 100); The Volvo Centre of Albemarle Street, London for the Volvo 245 DL Estate; Staples & Co Ltd for the bed; Wm Whitely Ltd for blankets; Brodie Sports for the shorts; Anthony Crickmay for the photograph of dancers and Runyon Associates of Vail, Colorado for the Skiers.

Most of the modelling was by Agape Stassinopoulos, Evelyne Duval and Malcolm Stoddard.

INDEX

Other recently published health books:

STRESS AND RELAXATION
Jane Madders, Dip Phys Ed, MCSP

Simple self-help methods of relaxation for anywhere and anytime. Once you know what relaxation is, you'll feel a different person.

DON'T FORGET FIBRE IN YOUR DIET
Denis Burkitt, MD, FRCS, FRS

This world-renowned medical scientist presents the first wide-ranging survey on the importance of fibre in preventing many typically western diseases.

BEAT HEART DISEASE!
Risteard Mulcahy, FRCPI, FRCP, MD

A reassuring look at one of today's most serious 'epidemics' – showing how changes in lifestyle could dramatically reduce the occurrence of heart disease and stroke.

OVERCOMING ARTHRITIS
Frank Dudley Hart, MD, FRCP

A leading rheumatologist describes just what arthritis and rheumatism are, and includes a wealth of ideas on how to keep your joints as supple and pain-free as possible.

ASTHMA AND HAY FEVER
Allan Knight, BSc, MD, CM, FRCP(C), FACP

Breathing difficulties or a streaming nose afflict thousands every year. Here an expert allergist explains what is happening to you and what you can do to ease the problems.

PSORIASIS
Prof Ronald Marks

An essential book for psoriasis sufferers, their families and all those with a professional interest in the condition.

MIGRAINE AND HEADACHES
Dr Marcia Wilkinson

An eminent migraine clinic director shows how to avoid and control the pain.

CONQUERING PAIN
Sampson Lipton, MB Ch B, DARCS(Eng) FFARCS(Eng)

Whether it's an arthritic joint, an excruciating backache, a throbbing migraine, this eminent pain-relief specialist provides reliable and straightforward information to help you understand, avoid and overcome the pain.

HIGH BLOOD PRESSURE
Dr Eoin O'Brien and Prof Kevin O'Malley

A comprehensive and practical guide to detecting, preventing and controlling one of the greatest risks to health and life expectancy.

THE HIGH-FIBRE COOKBOOK
Pamela Westland. Introduced by Dr Denis Burkitt

Over 200 delicious, tried and tested high-fibre dishes to help you eat well and stay healthy. Each recipe is accompanied by calorie, fibre and fat values.

THE DIABETICS' DIET BOOK
Dr Jim Mann and the Oxford Dietetic Group

The first book for diabetics and their dietitians that shows how to change to the new high carbohydrate and fibre diet now recommended by leading diabetic organizations around the world. Features over 140 mouthwatering recipes with full nutritional analyses.

DIABETES
Dr James Anderson

A complete new guide to healthy living for diabetics, featuring the recently developed high carbohydrate and fibre (HCF) diet programme.

VARICOSE VEINS
Prof Harold Ellis

A leading surgeon explains all the available treatments, and what you can do to help make them a success.

GET A BETTER NIGHT'S SLEEP
Prof Ian Oswald and Dr Kirstine Adam

These eminent sleep researchers give practical, scientifically based advice on how to avoid sleeplessness and wake refreshed every morning.

ECZEMA AND DERMATITIS
Prof Rona Mackie

Professor of Dermatology Rona Mackie sets out the facts about this ailment in down to earth, reassuring terms, and gives clear guidelines on what you should do to promote successful treatment.

ENJOY SEX IN THE MIDDLE YEARS
Christine Sandford, MD MRCS(Eng) LRCP(Lond)

As Marriage Guidance counsellor and adviser on sexual difficulties for over twenty years, Christine Sandford is well experienced in dealing with worries that get in the way of a smooth, harmonious love life.